D1760815

Materialist
Film

UNIVERSITY OF WESTMINSTER

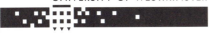

Materialist Film

Peter Gidal

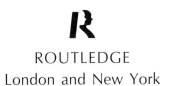

ROUTLEDGE

London and New York

First published in 1989 by
Routledge
11 New Fetter Lane, London EC4P 4EE
29 West 35th Street, New York NY 10001

Typeset by Columns of Reading
Printed in Great Britain
by TJ Press (Padstow) Ltd, Padstow, Cornwall.

British Library Cataloguing in Publication Data

Gidal, Peter
    Materialist film.
    1. Experimental cinema films
    I. Title
    791.43

Library of Congress Cataloguing in Publication Data

Gidal, Peter.
    Materialist film / Peter Gidal.
        p.   cm.
    Bibliography: p.
    Includes index.
    ISBN 0–415–00382–2 (pbk.)
    1. Experimental films—History of criticism.
    I. Title.
    PN1995.9.E96G53 1989

    791.43′01—dc19   88–15705
                               CIP

ISBN 0–415–00382–2

For Thérèse Oulton
every thought, thought through

We stood still to see the other cleft of Malebolge
and the other vain lamentings; and I found
it marvellously dark.

(Dante, *The Inferno*)

When you say experimental film is about trying to
understand the relationship between an object (in
this case an image) and its name, how we come to
know what we see, questioning the division of
reality into discrete entities, what are you questioning
about images? Images are not concepts, so how
does one go about questioning them?

(Christine Delphy, Interview with
Lisa Cartwright, *Undercut*)

Everything is optics.

(Nietzsche, *Complete Letters*)

Contents

Acknowledgements

I owe an inestimable debt to Philippa Brewster who commissioned this book.

Special thanks are due to the filmmakers and theorists who have allowed such extensive quotation. Malcolm LeGrice, Lis Rhodes, Deke Dusinberre, Lisa Cartwright, Stephen Heath, Nancy Woods, and Mike Dunford deserve singling out. I am particularly grateful to Malcolm LeGrice for his generosity of spirit since 1968.

The stills are all published here courtesy of the filmmakers, whom I thank also for in many cases spending time and effort to print good photos.

I am grateful to David Curtis for allowing untrammelled rifling though his archives.

Without the continual work at, and of, the London Filmmakers Co-operative, no British experimental film since 1966 would have been possible. And there is currently a presence there of a dozen important new filmmakers whose films will have their effects in the 1990s. My thanks to the Film Co-op are beyond measure.

Illustrations

Introduction

This book intends to theorize materialist film. It tries to utilize concepts that have been developed this century, in the interests of experimental filmmaking and thought. In doing so, it necessarily polemicizes certain positions and attempts to bring out specific uses in film, with the help of certain works of the avant-garde. The political positioning of the viewer is crucial in this, as is the knowledge that representation is real, is material, is politics and ideology, ideology the politics of meanings. Without a theory and practice of radically materialist experimental film, cinema would endlessly be the "natural" reproduction of capitalist and patriarchal forms.

I attempt in what follows to elucidate a series of concepts, tied to specific films in many cases, in a way that should allow the reader, by the time the book has been read, to deal with the issues and problematics that are produced by a materialist film theory and practice. None of this shall be without its problems.

The structure of the text is in "chapters," but the chapters do not somehow "lead" seamlessly towards a conclusion. Instead, a series of concepts are dealt with point for point, and the "order" is simply one that may allow the reader to make some relations. To present such a series of examinations as if they were "chronological" or "logical" or empirically related in a temporal manner would be simply to academicize the exercise towards the illusion of fulfillment. This would go against the meaning of the project. If anything, the series of adumbrations must be utilized not via some "pure objectivity" of knowing and not via some notion of individual subjectivity's truth. And certainly not via some "free" and "democratic" series of possibilities. Rather, bear in mind that the concepts do not appear in a vacuum, nor stem from one. It is a matter of things and concepts in constant dialectic material struggle in certain interests. How they are used is another matter.

Looking through the Table of Contents ought to give an immediate insight into the obviousness of what has been written so far.

I am using many long quotes in this text; the reason is that paraphrasing is tedious for reader and writer, and paraphrasing manages to take what polemical/theoretical/political power there is in writings and make it (them) somehow "part of" something else. Instead, these chapters (hopefully) engage with many of the meanings that are "quoted" or simply allow their force to persist. This may demand that the reader puts up with some difficulties in the process of reading/thinking, which is as things should be (and are).

My editor has written that parts of the book are like moving into, and then out of, a benign fog. I would merely add, not so benign.

I also hope that the readers do not find undue difficulties with the way this book is structured; it seems that all anthologies of film critical and film theoretical texts attempt one thing which this book does not: to have a variety of, strongly contradictory, texts sit happily side by side, something bourgeois academia and scholarship needs to survive. Survive it mustn't. It is no coincidence that film scholarship is as dull and as politically retrograde as sociology. Aesthetics have simply become comfortable, with a bit of Left-wing good conscience stuff added on to make the stultifying of convention appropriate and appropriated under the (incorrect) rubric of socialism (in England) and the (unfortunately correct) rubric of libertarianism (in the USA). In France the two are simply muddled together. It's all a sorry mess.

Would that much of what has been conceptualized in this book is of use and value to readers interested in experimental film, in the political ideology of viewing, in "cinema as such."

Some of the writings quoted engage my own films and writings. Some of the book is based on essays of mine published between 1968 and 1986, though many reworkings make the "original" unfindable in all this except when the source is given. Many polemical engagements with other theoreticians and filmmakers have led to countless reworkings so that a thought's origin (and originator) can not be conjured up. I hope some of my thoughts have become as lost in others' as theirs have in mine.

By the time the reader has finished with this book, he or she will hopefully have the wherewithal, partially from the reading itself, to engage with the materials of advanced film-practice. The latter, defined as experimental or avant-garde, means that a practice has specific currents and effects wherein contradictions are come upon forcing new threads of effect, both subjective and objective, which cannot be known and controlled in advance. No teleology ("toward . . .") must be inferrable. Thus experimental materialist film and film theory *make* politico-aesthetic history and ideology, both material.

Whether this is, or is not, a very good book, is not the main issue, if it produces positions of necessary conflict. So I hope the reader is armed with that thought, to no ill effect.

Many films have not been mentioned. Through ignorance and design, I have used examples that I know well, rather than allowing many more films to be cited in this or that section. Inevitably *Materialist Film* may look like some hierarchical list, all denials read as pro forma mea culpas. But of necessity the importantly determining works which are needed at each period for a practice to be sustainable do not all become isolable as exemplars, even though they may have been productive to the point of other works not having been possible without them! Such a double negative is their place in, or outside of, history, and currently all aesthetic practices operate in like manner. It stands to reason that in a different politico-aesthetic culture this would not be so.

1 The one to one relation between viewer and viewed

This concept of a one to one relation means that there is a direct analog between the represented film-time and the time for the viewer in the viewing-context. Such a relation can be set up in the most complexly edited film or in the simplest "single take." When complex editing is *not* used for the purposes of the seamless narrative continuum of classical narrative and its time-compressions, such complex editing can produce the "piece of time," time-fragments, that a one to one relation between viewer and viewed would demand. A common misunderstanding for the past two decades has been that avant-garde film fetishized this one to one relation, in a way which presupposed endless films made up of simple unedited shots. The same misunderstanding applied in respect of Warhol's work. In the latter case it took the critical form of describing loop-repeat shots, lasting two and a half minutes, as "seven-hour shots."[1] In general, in Britain, film theory made the assumptions that "British experimental film and structural/materialist film in particular, has relinquished editing" (*Screen*, 1978, Summer "Editorial").

Duration can be produced in various ways in experimental film, none of which necessitate denial of editing, and none of which posit a positivistic one to one relation between a continuum of time here and a continuum of time *there* (on screen, in frame). But there remains a problem, within the very *concept* of durational equivalence between shooting time and viewing time.

1

"Important to the presentation of process is an attention to temporality, as time is film's primary dimension (I would say material), and attention to duration (how long something lasts). It is usual in this connection to begin by adducing the exposition of the possible one to one relationship between shooting time and reading time, adducing an equivalence between the duration of the event recorded and the duration of the film representation of that event. A film such as *Couch* (Warhol, 1964) provides a stock example, with its takes the length of single rolls of film that are then joined together in sequence, this giving a shallow time which permits a credible relationship between the time of interior action and the physical experience of the film as a material presentation . . . which is Warhol's most significant innovation" (Malcolm LeGrice, *After Image*, no. 7, London 1978, p. 121).

LeGrice, for whom durational *equivalence* often seemed to be a primary ethic of filmmaking, found Michael Snow's *Wavelength* (1967) (see photograph on p. 157) seriously wanting on that score: "The one to one relationship between the projection duration and the shooting duration is lost through breaks in the shooting, not made clear in the form of the film. By utilizing a contrived continuity to parallel the implied time of its narrative, the film is in some ways a retrograde step in cinematic form" (ibid.).

Durational equivalence, however, is itself a turning back in cinema's history. It can function perfectly well, as the historical reception of the Lumiere films around 1910 demonstrates, as a foundation of the supreme illusion of the real, the actual "before one's eyes," so that according to Stephen Heath, "much more is at stake in Structural/Materialist film in the films themselves. The contrary practice of Structural/Materialist film is to break given terms of unity, to explore the heterogeneity of film in process. Snow's *Standard Time* (1967) for instance cites one reference (one standard) for time on the soundtrack, a morning radio broadcast, another on the imagetrack, an extremely elliptical human presence which conventionally, though not here, serves as the centre for the elision of the process of film-production, and here works over an eight minute duration of film with an unbound series of pans and tilts that ceaselessly pose the question of viewing time" (Stephen Heath,

"Notes around structural/materialist film," *Questions of Cinema*, Macmillan, 1981, London, and University of Indiana Press, 1981 and 1985).

What is defined by LeGrice as retrogression is *Wavelength's*, and any film's, construction which denies a temporal continuum. Where there is an edit, a cut, it must not be hidden. The complexity of commercial narrative cinema's editing techniques is precisely to efface the marks of the editing splice. Editing in the interests of the seamless flow of narrative utilizes a series of codes which demands a great deal of cutting, in the interests of the *effacement* of that process. To cite another example from LeGrice (from 1971), a sufficient lack of light ten minutes into a thirty-minute experimental film can function as an illusionistic *representation of a splice*, by functioning to mask the cut in the way other codes in conventional narrative cinema are utilized to mask this device. Thus LeGrice is demanding an anti-illusionist film practice polemically theorized in the interests of advanced, dialectical, experimental film. Such a position does not allow the surface "look" of an avant-garde film to somehow escape as rigorous a critique as dominant cinema. This position since the early 1960s has separated British experimental film-work from North American, which continually relied and relies on surface stylistic aspects for its self-definition. LeGrice's theorizing around film-practice had as its object the production of film-work which refused to allow the processes of filmmaking to become obliterated by, and subservient to, an overriding structural shape or aesthetic form. As such, a radically anti-bourgeois polemic was engaged, which the predominant North American writings on the avant-garde found themselves in opposition to. In film theory and practice as elsewhere, the danger for the British has always been empiricism, that for the Americans positivism; for the British, a radical negativity resulted nevertheless, for the Americans, an idealist positivity.

In North American film-writing, Warhol's *Chelsea Girls* (1966) and Snow's *Wavelength* (1967) have been defined in ways that obliterate their radically materialist processes. The latter for example is seen as "a grande metaphor for narrative," thereby obliterating the viewer's conscious and unconscious position in the cinematic process (Annette Michelson, *Artforum*, "Forward

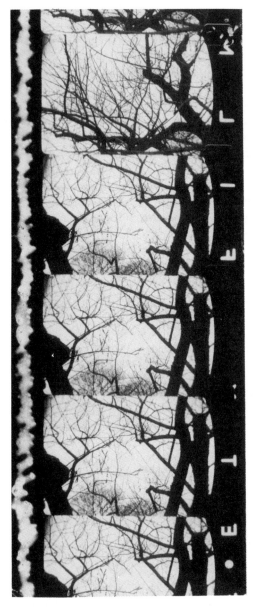

1 Kurt Kren, *Trees in Autumn* (1960)

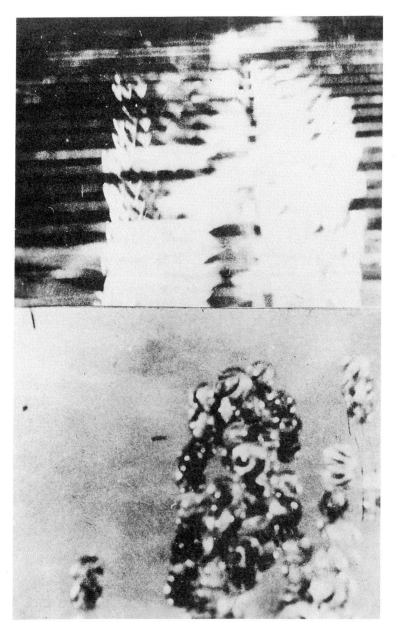

2 Germaine Dulac, *Étude Cinématographique sur une Arabesque* (1929)

in three letters" September 1971). By fetishizing surface *form*, bourgeois criticism intends the annihilation of materiality, and of social contradictions which imbricate the viewer. Bourgeois criticism equally intends annihilating the specific cinematic structures and histories engaged by a particular work. The dangers of an automatic temporal equivalence between film-time and viewing time in the "one to one relation of viewer and viewed" was continually dealt with in British filmmaking and writing, in order to use what was useful in such a durational equivalence. This led to the notion of pieces of material film-time as *not* being obliterated by illusionistic editing techniques, yet freed of the positivistic and mechanistic aspects. A series of quick cuts resulting in short bursts of half-second film movements, in Kurt Kren's *Trees in Autumn* (*Bäume im Herbst*) (Austria, 1960) can instigate a specific one to one relation rather than becoming a variegated jumble of images or an impressionistic haze. But such a process as in this film forces the viewer to make of the *possible* jumble of images discreet and separate segments. The process of the film demands a disruption of the "normal" cultural codes of viewing. Each shot becomes analysed and examined during the viewing, simultaneous to the moment to moment shock of each succeeding half-second "flash."

Trees in Autumn is a series of shots, each shot a density of trees and branches, the rhythm of the montage combined with the rhythm of movement or stillness with*in* each shot dominating any inferences (narrative or otherwise) from the represented space. This is also because the speed of shot following shot at half-second bursts flattens out the represented spaces seen. The relations of this film are shot-to-shot, rather than any internal editing complexities. A shot becomes a piece of time. A montage of shots in every film is a construction of duration and continuance in the face of the viewer's attempts to grasp and arrest the seen, attempts at making definition and meaning. When the film at hand refuses to fill those meanings with "truth" or "nature" or "the real," meanings are unmade as quickly as made. The viewer is positioned to expect certain things, and to expect to be able to proceed with certain meanings (let's say about "nature" when seeing "trees" represented). The artifice and ideology of meaning is a process that can be constantly problematized in the realm, amongst others, of film. Representation matters, it is realism of another kind. A materialist experimental film practice engages on that level with the illusions of representation and the illusory (and real!) constructs of viewing film, or anything, as if it were natural.

Through such acts of perception, a new object results.[2] This "object" is a process, the process of materialist film. Yet this must not be understood to mean that the manner of viewing *creates* the object. What it means is that the film material and the process of viewing together transform film into a new object and process. Filmic "trying to see" instead of seeing, trying to know instead of (the illusion of) knowing. Not believing what is seen.

The notion of post-Eisensteinian editing, with, for example, parallel montage (two things going on in different places at the same time, building suspense) is fundamentally opposed to film-as-duration as previously described. But the danger of such a concept is that it limits "Eisensteinian editing" to the Eisenstein *form* of editing, as if that were mechanically applicable to any scenario, or film idea, or bit of film. It also does not take account of the strategies of editing in his early work *Strike* (1924) in which the techniques of montage (of collision) produced filmic montage-as-duration, the foregrounded setting up of artifice and form within structures *not* subsumed by narrative. This was why Eisenstein at the time was accused of formalism! Kren's film is based on mathematical structures, which are utilized to montage the film, to systematize its "putting together." But such a construct has nothing to do with any *effect* of "discovering structure" via viewing. It is a crucial misunderstanding of the notion of structure that led to the definitions of Structural Film in the United States in the late 1960s to mean a film wherein "the overall shape predominates" (P. A. Sitney, "Structural film," *Film Culture Reader*, New York, 1969). Such overall shape was seen to take precedence both over the functions within any internal segments and equally over all filmic processes. The viewer, viewer-as-subject, is left out completely as well, as the object for consumption in such an aesthetic, and its notions of the artist/auteur/voyeur, hardly differed from that of the ideologies of commercial narrative film. One does not read out the structure from *Trees in Autumn*, or puzzle together the elements. One does attempt to decipher constantly. To decipher what? The workings and transformations of the process of representation, the forms produced, the contradictions of filmmaking subjectivity in relation to "representing the world;" all the latter are effects of specific usages. These inculcated attempts to decipher have to do with representation and repetition. Each film segment places itself both with and against the preceding and following, thereby disallowing any easy flow of the cinematic. Making difficult is one aesthetic process here. The question of *anything* being held, finalized, stopped, is constantly problematic in such a film. No more the illusion of the end of movement produced *by* the movements of time and image. The relation of such structural/materialist films as *Trees in Autumn* and *Yes No Maybe Maybe Not* (LeGrice, 1967, see discussion on p. 124) to structuralist activity in other fields is obvious, and also problematic.

Film-works can produce an analytic situation in the very processes of their procedure, not as an academic afterthought, not as analysis *versus* film-as-projected. If analysis is thus not interpretation/analysis-after-the-fact, then it is not a time-denying process, and the questions of memory and constant rememoration attempts, during viewing, become paramount.

"The first embodiment of this concept of structural activity in cinema comes in Kren's *Bäume im Herbst* where the camera as subjective observer is constrained within a systemic or structural procedure, incidentally the precursor of the most structuralist aspect of Michael Snow's later work. In this film, perception of material relationships . . . is seen to be no more than a product of the structural activity in the work. Barthes echoes this 'no more than' and says of it: 'this appears to be little enough, which make some say the structuralist enterprise is meaningless, uninteresting, useless, etc. Yet from another point of view, this "little enough" is decisive. There appears something new' " (LeGrice, quoting Barthes).

This is not the place or time to critique LeGrice's positions for their adherence to an existential stance, albeit coterminal with the materialist positions taken up. An epistemological break (Althusser) is necessary for certain positions to exist and have their use, though practice is often ahead of theory, and one always speaks in "the old language." *Post*-existential avant-garde/experimental film has persisted in Britain since

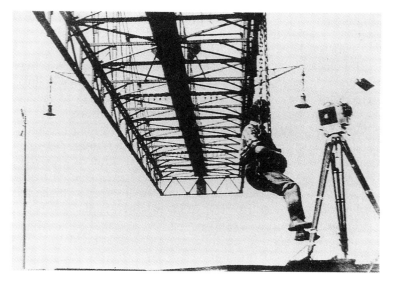

3 Dziga Vertov, *The Man with the Movie Camera* (1928/9)

1966, not coincidentally vouchsafed by LeGrice's film of 1967 *Yes No Maybe Maybe Not.*

This is being written at a time of a rightwing, and equally dangerous libertarian, backlash in the arts, in sexuality, in the economy, in cultural–political meanings. Yet some aspects of Marxism and, more importantly, radically materialist feminism, have remained rigorous about current necessities. The contradictory histories of subjectivity within a materialist aesthetic must occur without the reactionary existential, expressionist and neo-expressionist, romantic and neo-romantic, politic.

"Kren's first structuralist film is 3/60–*Bäume im Herbst* (3/60 being Kren's numbering system). The first film in general that I would call Structuralist. Its structuralism is a result of the application of system, not to subsequent montage of material already filmed with an unconstrained subjectivity, but to the act and event of filming itself. This limitation, by narrowing the space and time range of the shot material, gives rise to greater integrity in the film as homologue (integrity as clinical description, not ethical norm). In *Bäume im Herbst* the new space/time fusion of the experience of branches shot against the sky IS the plasticity of the shooting system become the relations of the objects. Shots, and their space/time observational *relations*, are inseparable" (Malcolm LeGrice, "Kurt Kren's films," *Studio International*, Film Issue, November 1975, p. 187).[3]

The closest precursor to this would be Rodchenko's photographs in the 1920s in the Soviet Union, and the angular disorientation of some of the photojournalistic work of the late 1920s in Europe, particularly in Germany.

Germaine Dulac's *Arabesque* (1929) is the stunning precursor in film of such work. She writes: "When the idea of abstract cinema, which is expressed by the visual rendering of pure movement beyond the existing aesthetics, is presented to the greater part of the public and even to many intellectuals and professional filmmakers, it is received with scepticism, if not open hostility; it is allowed to evolve provided that in its striving for perfection this new art movement does not break with the formal framework of tradition.

"But suddenly from various points of the globe dedicated filmmakers, without knowing or having any contact with each other, isolated in the silence of their thoughts and intuitions while following the same line of research, have converged at the same frontier.

"Abstract . . . cinema should not therefore be derided or held suspect since with the constructive energy of some and in its already significant appeal to a few others, it exists by virtue of that very fact. Conceived, wished for, and already concretely formulated in several works, it has progressed from the limbo of nebulous theories into the material domain of expression.

"But soon it seemed to me that the expressive value of a fact was contained less in the general aspect of the features themselves than in the mathematical duration of their reactions.

"Followers . . . are treated as utopians. Why? For myself, I'm not arguing the need for emotive values in the concept of a work. The creative will should reach the public's understanding through the conscious theme which unites them. But what I oppose is the narrow interpretation which is generally made of movement. Because movement and rhythm remain. . ." (Germaine Dulac, 1927, "Du Sentiment a la ligne" [Sentiment by the yard], in the journal *Schemas*).

Arabesque and *Trees in Autumn*: a historical process exists in the viewing of such work, or, the historical process of viewing is not suppressed/repressed in such work. The social discourse of experimental cinema is instituted in this way, against the individualist discourse of the sometimes seemingly more social existence of dominant cinema. The importance of the history of each viewing is inseparable from the subject/viewer's own history but not somehow determined by it. This gives the material of film power through which the cinematic event persists. It is in the manner described above that the shorthand "one to one relation of viewer to viewed" must be understood.

2 The concept of arbitrariness

The concept of "arbitrariness" is based on the political demand that nothing be accepted as natural. This is not a denial of meanings but rather a recognition of the imposition of ideologies. Anything that smacks of essence or the pregiven is inimical to a materialist aesthetic politics. Religion similarly. In film, as in all representational practices, various discourses clash. There is a political conflict. And forms clash as they are political meanings, are in political conflict both *as* meaning and *for* the meanings they "contain."

The "arbitrary" is a concrete concept which is embattled, in relation to concepts such as "essence" and "nature" and the pregiven. "Arbitrariness" in sound and image *each moment* goes against granting a *fullness* to an image moment. Arbitrariness and the constructedness of each image–sound conjunction and disjunction must be produced by (in) the film, a film–viewer relation. Each "image moment" thus does not mean a moment of "fullness", it merely designates *moment*, not static, not essential, not somehow quintessentially ontologically "filmic," simply a clinical description of a moment or piece of time. A rejection of any metaphysic is therefore emphasized here, otherwise a phrase such as "image moment," even within a description of the materialist concept "arbitrariness," could reinveigle itself as a metaphysic of film. This would be precisely the opposite of what a materialist defining and theorizing has for its object and impetus.

The notion of arbitrariness links to the concept of the empty signifier, the *attempted* (always failed) construction of such a signifier towards *non-identity*. Thus the self-identity that is constantly reproduced in illusionist representations and the consequent positions of the viewer in his/her unconscious identities, according to the dominantly reproduced models of sex, class, race, is in opposition to a materialist practice which attempts the constant construction of non-identity. This is a break from infinitude and eternity, which a religiously capitalist patriarchy attempts to designate and reproduce. Such imperialisms are dominant and in certain interests. The construction of non-identity in the filmic process attempts to radicalize the conscious and unconscious positioning of the viewer/listener. One lineage from the work of Gertrude Stein and Samuel Beckett can be acknowledged.

What French radical feminist Christine Delphy polemicizes is, for this matter of gender identity, precise: "Another problem is that women who have relationships with men can only go so far and they then have to stop or they couldn't live with the idea. They couldn't go on sleeping with men. And they have to go on sleeping with men, for all sorts of reasons (they can't be blamed for that) because they're constructed that way. Well, let's not say that; *we're* constructed that way. But in any case it becomes an unbearable contradiction if you take it to its logical conclusion. Because then you start questioning everything you do and you can't go on living. Heterosexuality as a sort of cosmic heterosexuality is absolutely coterminal with a basic world view which not only hasn't been put into question, but if it were put into question everything would crumble down . . . nobody would know who they are.

"You can call into question your class and ethnic identification without eliminating your sense of self. But if people are not men and women anymore, then they don't know who they are. No identity. It's not a personal problem of not having any other identity. The problem is that no other personal identity (identities) exists, because identity is built on gender identity. Attacking sexuality . . . is in the end attacking the assumption that men and women are complementary somehow, at some very basic level. And that basic level is represented by coitus. When one questions that, one questions everyone's identity. People cannot afford to be left without an identity, so we cannot approach a question that might lead to that" (Christine Delphy, "Interview with Laura Cottingham," *Off Our Backs*, August 1984.)

She hereby does approach this question! "It is a contradiction, for instance, when we use the word 'women' and we don't agree with the category 'women'. In the first editorial statement in *Questions Feministes* (June 1977) we say that we are aiming for a world without sexual division. In this, the words 'men' and 'women' won't have meaning. People will be identified differently, not through that division" (Christine Delphy, " 'On representation and sexual division,' Interview with Lisa Cartwright," *Undercut*, nos. 14/15, Summer 1985.)

The problem for structural/materialist film is that the concepts of arbitrariness and non-identity can not be *simply* applied; each work has its specificities. There is no overall aesthetic strategy which assures certain results or effects. This is also the problem for post-structural/materialist film, "post" in the sense of what comes after and takes its lessons into account, not "post" as in "post-feminist," or "post-marxist," or "post-modernist" meaning to reject the radicality of the previous.

An example: most of the abstract color-field films of Paul Sharits (*Ray Gun Virus*, 1966; *T.O.U.C.H.I.N.G.*, 1968; *Axiomatic Granularity*, 1973) have a grainy, perspectively deep illusionism within which a conventional, and often reactionary, psychological identification process takes place. The level of abstraction is to the point of total abstract, within which, then, "paradoxically," the documentary truth of the represented film-grain becomes the dominant factor, the narrative even. Such depth produced through the abstract forms the instigations for viewing which foster imaginary identities for the viewer, identities which conventional narrative produces with narrative plot. The abstract, in the above example, operates this way by never existing in relation to representation, to the issues of representation. Thus no contradictions are set up which would instigate a critical process of difficulty between the seen and the meanings inculcated, or the seen in relation to what the viewer

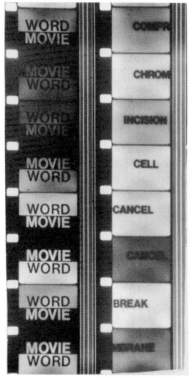

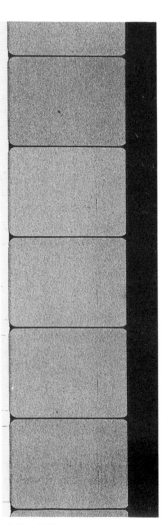

4 Paul Sharits, *Word Movie* (1966)

5 Paul Sharits, *Axiomatic Granularity* (1973)

thinks he/she "knows" as to the referential meanings. There is no dialectic between, for example, the momentary grasping at pregiven meanings and their being simultaneously undermined as well as produced *as* constructions. What is thus lacking is a blast of problematic at any one moment which could position a viewer very differently from comfortable abstract, "pure," light and grain. In the same sense, an abstract painting is not more *a priori* against identification than a non-abstract one. Popova's *Spatial Force Construction* (1920), Kandinksy's 1914 period abstract paintings, Klee's *2nd Part of Poem by Wang Seng Yu* (1916), Rozanova's *Book Cover* (Needlework, 1916), Stella's Black Paintings (1959) must be differentiated from, for example, the imaginary identity-production of Picasso, Rothko. This is roughly stated as a particular work can be in radical opposition to another work by the same artist. The willed analysis which puts an abstract Sharits film into some kind of radical formal category based on its surface look in crude positivistic opposition to dominant narrative cinema is a bourgeois formalism which reproduces dominant conventions all the more categorically. It is not coincidental that such positions largely occurred in the United States. "I am an illusionist. I am into illusionism" (Paul Sharits, "Statement", Buffalo, N.Y, 1976).

To add confusion to the issue, the Sharits films named and alluded to have intercut sections of straightforward psychodramatic narrative moments, all the more making metaphor out of the filmic usages of "pure" color, light, grain; all the more an anti-materialist project. Yet *Word Movie* (1966) elegantly and powerfully problematizes language and image illusion.

3 Implicating materialism with physicality

The concept of materialism cannot be covered by the concept and concrete reality of physicality. The attempt here is by fits and starts to elucidate a materialist process. The questions pertaining to representation-systems and codes has to do with the *physical* reproduction and transformation of *forms*, a reproduction, at some level, of the profilmic, that which the camera is aimed at – a transformation *to* the filmic, the filmic event, so to speak. This transformation has to do with codes of cinematic usage which for the most part are not yet clearly delineated in the case of experimental film. For example, there is no questioning that the dissolution of imagery through extremes of darkness and light also (and equally) has to do with the flattening of the screen-surface, bringing that screen-surface-ness into play against the (however momentarily) held depth-illusions, i.e. representation of the real world via cinematic photochemical means. It is thus unquestionable that a certain usage of grain and contrast can produce itself *vis à vis*, and through, the *image*. The duration of that "image," and that image's transformation, always preceded by other images, always effecting other images, and their meanings and uses, is inseparable from the material–physical support. This is in no way to say that what is materialist in film is what necessarily *shows*, or that it is camera, lenses, graininess, flicker *per se*, etc. But an idealist negation of physicality *in toto* can only lead to a blindness.

"I felt *Room Film 1973* was made by a blind man, trying to see" (Michael Snow, Statement, September 1973, NFT, London).

4   Presence

Filmic presence must mean present operations and processes, in distinction to *usage*, usage towards some other ends. Presence as immanence is opposed to presence as dialectical. Where then is Derrida's presence?: "We shall designate by the term differance (with an 'a') the movement by which language or any code, any system of reference in general, becomes historically constituted as a fabric of differences. *Differance* is what makes the movement of signification possible only if each element is said to be "present," appearing on the stage of "presence," is related to something other than itself, but retains the mark of a past element and already lets itself be hollowed out by the mark of its relation to a future element. This trace relates no less to what is called the future than to what is called the past, and it constitutes what is called the present by this very relation to what it is not, to what it absolutely is not; that is, not even to a past or future considered as a modified present. . . . We ordinarily say that a sign is put in place by the thing itself, the present-thing, "thing" holding here for the sense as well as the referent. Signs represent the present in its absence; they take the place of the present. When we cannot take hold of or show the thing, let us say the present, the being present, when the present does not present itself, *then* we signify, we go through the detour of signs" (Jacques Derrida, "Differance," *Speech and Phenomena*, Northwestern University Press, 1973, quoted in "Theory and definition of structural/materialist film," *Studio International*, November 1975, p. 191). Such concepts were worked through filmically in certain London Filmmakers Co-op films long before Derrida verbalized them, but such verbalization clarifies certain aspects of the problematic by bringing it to speech. Just as there is a split between filmic and verbal articulation, there is a split in the viewing, which is why Derrida and post-structuralist critics, whether of the Left or Right, have an exceedingly hard time watching, and engaging with, such filmwork. Practice becomes impossible, *possible only in language after the fact*. Such splits are inevitable, so that political and philosphical theory, and theorists, lag in terms of filmic cultural political practice. (Only one philosophy acknowledges that all histories are dialectically materialist.)

A film is materialist if it does not cover its apparatus of illusionism. Thus it is not a matter of anti-illusionism pure and simple, uncovered truth, but rather, a constant procedural work against the attempts at producing an illusionist continuum's hegemony. Anti-illusionist materialist cinema is one which does not give the illusion of having dispensed with such questions. But such work, simultaneously, is not just a defensive practice against some hegemonic given against which it must constantly rail; it is not only in opposition, revolutionary, which would be enough. It equally forcefully has its own history, another history, which only bourgeois "history" suppresses. Other histories than the dominant ones exist in every discourse, the politics of representation being not the least of these.

As everything is materialist, this is both a strength of all processes and discourses, and a problem. The problem is that anyone can choose any "good object" and critique it, interpret it, by bringing out "what it is *really* doing." Thus, analysis of one's preferred object, whether it be *Gilda* or *Touch of Evil* or *The Birds* or *Gertrud* or some Godard film or *Thriller* or *Jeanne Dielman* or *Daughter Rite* or *Born in Flames* resuscitates the object, reproduces its positions even if analysis is critical, demands it as good object of desire even when, and in fact precisely when, contradictions are brought out. In that way, academic discourse solidifies the status quo of power and authority whilst ostensibly positioning itself (sometimes) against it. Such fetishized authorizations for interpretation of the viewed are fundamentally conservative *in structure*.

5 Content

The content serves as a function upon which, time and time again, a filmmaker works to bring forth the filmic event. "Function upon which" must be understood as a function *through* which, not as overlayering.

6 The subject

Some work is beginning to be done on the production of meaning and constitution of the viewer-as-subject. Important is the concept of a non-static, not memory-less, viewer. Important is that the view*ing* is not of a stasis designated the film. This leads all the way to ideology as not a covering which you take off (or pull off!) only to find unveiled certain meanings.

There can be a danger with too emphatic a notion of the constant building/construction of a subject/viewer which, misinterpreted, *misunderstood*, could lead to notions of constant renewal, consciousness force-feeding, *person* as completely ahistorically formed. A history exists for each subject, as does memory and attempted rememoration, subject-construction and the necessary critique against any *unified* self. Investigation along these lines may be of importance to advanced film-practice as well as to reactionary film-practice.

In all the above what must be resisted is the imposition of an idea of "the context" in any way which would give itself a power to overdetermine the material (film) at hand/to eye. The realization must be that the "I" is both produced by, and producing. It is neither a simple "Individual consciousness makes the world" nor a straightforward "Social relations produce consciousness, produce the I." Reinstigated is the power of individualism when the term "context" is seen to cause and rationalize all interpretations of film, and its meanings and processes. Such a return to a pre-socialist politics of representation is dangerous in that it is done in the name of social(ist) discourse, as if the privileging of context means doing battle with a "vulgar materialism of the reified object," as if the privileging of context were doing battle with empiricist fallacies. When in fact *context* has been used against the *materiality of film, the materiality of filmic procedures*. As if by setting up false oppositions one could solve theoretical problems! Un-entanglement must take place here.

In the last two decades, those adhering to the *context*-side, or tendency, in this "debate" have done so and do so inarticulately, that is to say, they *identify*. The "context" position allows *any* interpretation to hold, rationalized via lit-crit sociologese. These identifications position certain filmmakers, critics, teachers, and have effects on filmwork and equally job opportunities, journalistic power, public sanction. This is a state of things detrimental to a working through and possible *reduction* of these complex issues. The context/material fissure finds itself here.

7 Film as film

This dangerous formulation of mine from 1971 was wrongly taken to mean that film's essential nature was the proper area of investigation for avant-garde/experimental film. It was never up to the structural/materialist filmmaker to recover films' essential nature, i.e. film as film. If anything, it is *a* film's concrete existence which must interest; its possibilities of militating against transparency; its presentation/formation of processes of production which have as their uses meanings constructed by, through, and *for*. In what interests are constructions constructed? Films can operate to produce their processes against imaginary constructions. Imaginary constructions are those whose components and meanings are not produced as obsessive, difficult, contradictory, because an uncontradictory *construction* is one that gives itself as natural. Not produced at all – out of the blue! That imaginary then becomes that area that *demands* narrative identification, ideological desires fulfilled, and so on.

The photochemical process can put an "imaginary" image on the screen; at the same time, a film-process can produce this imaginary *as imaginary*. Thus it is not a matter of "non-manipulative" cinema, but of an awareness of its manipulations in-process, not after the fact. Secondly, the photochemical imprint is not an illusion, it is a simple material, not materialist, process. It formulates a grained image in the emulsion of film, subsequently projected by a physical light beam onto a light surface, the screen.

Such formulations could lead LeGrice, for example in the late 1960s, to realize that a film in which a section goes so dark as to be nearly indecipherable may simultaneously demand of the viewer the will and need to see, to decipher. Unable to do so, to make active the viewer's perceptive processes, whilst simultaneously positioning him/her as *impossible* in relation to *any* "truth" of image. Representation as representation. Against this there are codes of naturalness, identification-mechanisms, which make the imaginary operate as real. LeGrice's insight was that lack of light could be representing the splice, "hidden in darkness," even if there was no empirical evidence. This critique was located at the level of possible illusionism within the ostensible anti-illusionist project of certain London Co-op Filmmakers' works (including my own). This critique set film*making* and its research-work, both theoretically and practically, one step forward. The articulation of theory of, for, and *as* film, is how such materialist experimental work operates, and operated at the London Film Co-op since 1967.

8 Perception versus knowledge

This is a complexity instilled by the materialist process of some works, whilst others give perception and the perceived the ideology of a oneness, the true, for the perceiver. Still others give truth as cinematically hidden from perception, alluded to from offscreen, implied, metaphorized. One way perception versus knowledge might be filmically constructed is stated in these notes from *Condition of Illusion* (1975): "This film is, in its viewing, a process that attempts to make sure of a retroactive reading, *whilst viewing*. Reading/viewing as knowledge, not immediate 'realization.' Not an *image* (of 'a splice' for example) but a knowledge (of 'that'). 'That' being textually functional/transformational, not static.

"The final print necessitated three internegatives which were edited together, a + b rolled expressly to suppress, as in dominant, conventional cinema, the connecting splices. The loop structure of the editing, though undermined by various camera tactics, brings forth (foregrounds) (to understanding) the presence (in absentia) of the connecting splices.

"Thus seeming continuity, as in dominant cinema. Discontinuities are brought out in the same way as above. Pieces of time, durational structures, assert themselves in retrospect, *during* the viewing-time, and *vis à vis* previous and anticipated segments. There are, for example, *similar shots*, different enough to seem at first dissimilar, therefore allowing continuity of time without interruption or repetition, *then* realized as in fact a re-take of the same. In this way the re-take is formulated not on some illusionist level of what could be called a crude materialist insight, wherein one would conceptualize that 're-take' as a mechanistic, empirical fact which the film *documents*. Conventional documentaries document; and fiction-narratives in that way 'recreate' whatever story it is they are telling.

"Loop structures in *Condition of Illusion* are not utilized as in loop structures pure and simple wherein there could be no seeming linearity or continuity. The imagery has to be different enough to enforce the possibility of a continuum onto something different, only then realized as the same.

"The lack of difficulty in seeing, in this film, i.e. the clarity, the quantity of light and focus, contrasts with my other main films and is meant to work in relation to the obvious, opaque, camera-technical usages, specifically: fast back and forward zooms; fast movement 'around' the space, without letting an imaginary space become built up for/through the viewer's desires for structured coherence and unity; abrupt movements, not blurring but annihilating image definition. There is, I think, a virtual and an actual inseparability of abstract from concrete the way the mechanisms have here been used to produce the image-shot-segments-whatever.

"The viewer must be in the position of not-knower. No construct of the offscreen space is adequately given. The fusion (any fusion constructed) is given as construct. Disfusion similarly. There is great difficulty in reading out any space from the film. In such filmic structurings arrestation and rememoration attempts constantly reposition the viewer in the split of knowledge versus perception, the known and believed thereby made unknown. This position of unknowing creates a position antagonistic to the dominant ideological operation of illusionist truth, and of meaning as pregiven to any labour process. The viewer is fractured from her/his superior position of consumer of knowledge, fractured from the illusion of power over the representation, fractured from full self identity, which are the prerequisites for narrative completion" (from "Notes on

Condition of Illusion," National Film Theatre, London 1975). It is important not to forget that such notes are always written long after the film is finished.

"In *Condition of Illusion*," according to Stephen Heath, "what is not achieved is the stabilization of reproduction into the terms of a representation: effectively, the materials of reproduction that are engaged by the film are not stabilized into representation; the photograph (for several seconds eight minutes into the film) given precisely as a holdable moment (why else a photograph if not for that?). The distinction between reproduction and representation is important, though difficult. In a sense, all films of Gidal's that I have seen are full of the materials of reproduction held off of – not fixed into – representation. Duration and narrative thus come apart, narrative being exactly fixing, stabilization. In the phrase 'reproduction of reality', reality itself means a specific set of reproductions, reproducible representations, positions, stabilities, clarities. Representation is a series of positions for the spectator in relation to a certain clarity of position and meaning" (Stephen Heath, "Cambridge tapes 1977," *The Cinematic Apparatus*, eds S. Heath and T. de Lauretis, Macmillan, London and St Martins Press, New York, 1981 and 1985, p. 165, n. 2).

"The disunity, the disjunction, of Structural/Materialist film is, exactly, the spectator. What is intended, what the practice addresses, is not a spectator as unified subject, timed by a narrative action, making the relations the film makes to be made, coming in the pleasure of the mastery of those relations, of the positioned view they offer, but a spectator, a spectating activity, at the limit of any fixed subjectivity, materially inconstant, dispersed in process, beyond the accommodation of reality and pleasure principles. . . . Of no one memory: in *Condition of Illusion*, the return of an impossible openness of the film as object of desire, flashes of memories, this statuette, this rapid zoom in and out, this white surface, this pulling of focus, a network in which the vision of the I, the ego, is no longer confirmed as the master view.

"In *Condition of Illusion*, which involves the instability of possibilities of recognition (speed of camera movement, use of focus, proximity, angle, etc, leaving only a few objects and

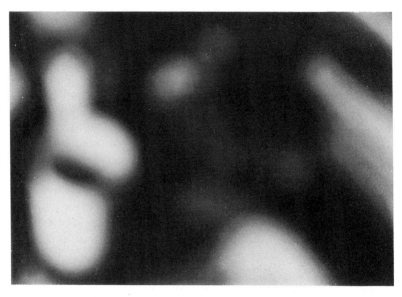

6 Peter Gidal, *4th Wall* (1978)

places in the room identifiable according to the norms of photographic reproduction), the repetition suggests a possibility of
'catching up', 'making sure', 'verifying', which in fact remains
unexploitable, ineffective (one never sees 'more'),[5] resistant in
the very literalness of the repetition (no variation, modulation,
no 'new angle').

"In general, Structural/Materialist films are engaged with
images, assume the fact of their production, and often attempt
to move in the time of that production. This is an effect of *Condition of Illusion* where camera focus and pace seem frequently
to be hesitating just on the boundary of stability and recognition.
Which is to say that Structural/Materialist films begin at least,
like any other type of film, from the primary identification that
Metz sees as constitutive in the cinematic apparatus itself: 'the
spectator identifies with him/herself as a pure act of perception
(as wakefulness, alertness), as condition of possibility of the
perceived and hence as a kind of transcendental subject. . . .
As he/she identifies with him/herself as look, the spectator can
do no other than identify with the camera too, which has looked

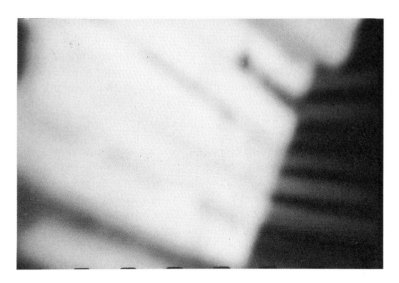

7 Peter Gidal, *Condition of Illusion* (1975)

before at what is now being looked at. . . .' They begin from but end against the solicitation of the unity of the look that the apparatus offers for exploitation, is developed to exploit: the all-perceiving subject free in the instrumentality of the camera that serves to relay and reproduce at every moment the power of that central vision. Structural/Materialist film has no *place* for the look, ceaselessly displaced, outphased, a problem of seeing; it is anti-voyeuristic" (Stephen Heath, "Repetition time: notes around structural/materialist film," in *Questions of Cinema*, Macmillan, London, and University of Indiana Press, 1981 and 1985, pp. 165–15).

"After a viewing of *Condition of Illusion*, the account given will be extremely 'subjective' (particular traces of the desiring relation, liking–remembering this or that moment, wanting it in the repetition), or extremely 'objective' (towards a description of the film's construction, its use of repetition, camera mobility, and so on), the two, exactly at their extreme, joining up with one another; what is missing is the habitual common ground, the narrative metaphor or transference or model of the film, its memory for the spectator placed as its subject, bound and centred on its terms of meaning. Or rather, the spectator as subject-ego (the ego is the place of the imaginary identifications of the subject), the maintained illusion of coherence (derived in film from the maintained coherence of the illusion); but the subject is always more than the ego, the 'more' that Structural/Materialist film seeks to open out in its demonstration of process" (ibid.).

Against that kind of critico-filmic position, an example of a film which looks stylistically "different" yet in that guise mimics the conventions of dominant cinema would be the Straub/Huillet film, *Introduction to the Accompaniment to a Cinematographic Scene by Arnold Schönberg* (also 1975). It offers an interesting example of a failure, not because it foregrounds problems of narrativity somehow – it does not – but because it posits notions of perfect narrative, in relation to letters sent between Kandinsky and Schönberg, suggestive of a perfect documentary. It even records the fact that some of the letters are missing, and employs black leader (spacing) as the perfect representation of an empty space – as if empty space could exist, and as if black leader could perfectly represent anything, save when used in an illusionist fashion.

Straub/Huillet and Godard serve mainly as examples against a materialist experimental avant-garde cinema, and have had their conflictual relations with it at levels of production, distribution, and exhibition in Britain, France, Germany, and the United States. As is evident in what follows.

"Jean-Marie does most of the talking. It was interesting to note that when it came to a long technical point-for-point detailing of how the sound-work was done, Danielle elaborated concretely each necessary item of information. Also, when there were things to be said filling in or redirecting Straub's statements, Danielle Huillet would, in a low voice, say them to him, not the audience. Obviously all this leads to speculation as to the specific roles taken, and to what degree there is real collective work. Certain points need discussing, if only because Straub/Huillet's positions both in speech and in the films were unfortunately influential ones. Straub/Huillet talked, for example, of splicing black leader into the film *Introduction to the Accompaniment* every time there was an elision, a cut, in the

Schönberg text being quoted. 'Every time you have a piece of black leader it is because we cut something out, and between these two Schönberg letters there is an answer by Kandinsky which we do not have anymore.' That Straub/Huillet should think that black leader as a replacement for something 'missing' is an adequate *filmic* solution places their theoretical stance into that of the *pseudo-documentary*. In other words, the film-work is seen by them as an adequate documentation of what is.

"The replacement of one thing (sentences from a letter, cut out) for another (black leader, spacing) tends to repress precisely the practice of filmmaking as a production. There is not, perfectly, a reproduction of an externally existent reality perfectly documentable through film. Though there is the illusion of such! (A notion of '*im*perfect documentation' would not subvert the concept of the pseudo-documentary, merely 'literalize' it, as if there were a perfect representation of documentary truth somehow not totally achieved at this instance or that.) A crisis existed in the avant-garde around 1975–80 which was relevant to the film-work of various British experimental filmmakers Malcolm LeGrice, Mike Dunford, William Raban associated with the Filmmakers Co-op and, on a much less sophisticated level, relevant to independent filmmakers working at the Royal College of Art and through the British Film Institute Production Board, whose work had, in varying degrees, found itself caught up inside this problem. For the replacement of a gap (missing letter, or section) by a segment of film (black or otherwise) sets up a replacement-duration which is in no way an attack on the concept and function of adequate and perfect/perfectable representation, either as documentary truth or fictional narrative.

"Another point about Straub/Huillet's apparent belief in adequate documentation is the usage in most of their films of a *pretext*. The problem of distanciation (engagement's inseparability from thought) is supposedly taken on. The concept of distanciation must never be understood as simple distancing. If a Schönberg piece (say *Moses and Aaron*) is used, the viewer must, constantly and from the beginning, be in the position of defining the degree of emotional distance from the text itself that the film is or is not achieving. This distanciation, if the film is not to become merely an adequate documentation of an opera performance, is crucial.

"*Moses and Aaron* is an opera in three acts: the first deals with the calling of Moses, his meeting with Aaron in the desert, and their announcement of the message of God to the people; in the second act Aaron, the Elders, and the People wait before the Mountain of Revelation for the return of Moses; the third act is Moses' condemnation of Aaron. With their terror of dubbing, the Straubs insisted that the singers should sing their parts on location, only the orchestra having been pre-recorded in Vienna. This terror of dubbing is understandable given German cinema's habit of dubbing everything into four-voice drivel, pastiche without knowing it. But to then mistheorize this for a concept of synchronization's 'greater truthfulness' is a confusion that becomes the other side of the (same) coin.

"One point Huillet raises is that of the actors'/singers' dual foci, to the director of the film and to the director of music, not to mention triple foci through the person being addressed. Now this dialectic tension which would indeed bring forth a Brechtian theatrico-filmic distanciation-construct, is, in *Moses and Aaron*, not evident in the finished film. In fact, the matter becomes more difficult because each singer has an earphone, and thus can only be filmed from one side. This too could lead to a kind of distanciation, if one were, as filmmaker, aware of the difference between intent and effect, and had a materialist process of production as one's basic aesthetic and political practice, rather than a humanistic–mystical/mystifying one. Ego, in the latter, overrides any material function that the apparatus has at any level, and the scene becomes, as in most cinema, a spectacularization of the artist's said ego, and the social conventions through which it functions. This is a basic tenet of humanist art. The viewer then receives the film, the film-text, acting, singing, in such a way that there is no reason to question at any moment the direction an actor/singer speaks or sings or gestures to. There is no difficulty with the directionality imposed by constraints of the apparatus, thus no dialectic resistence for the viewer via identifications engaged" (Peter Gidal, *Ark, Journal of the Royal College of Art*, 1976, p. 37–49).

The image is filled by the music, which is something current neo-romantic independent film of the mid 1980s has

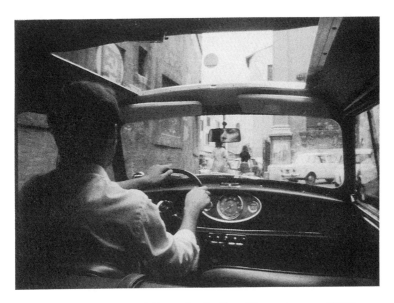

8 Jean-Marie Straub/Danielle Huillet, *History Lessons* (1974)

perpetuated (Derek Jarman, Cerith Wynn Evans, and others), obviously in very different ways; filling the image with sound has reached the apotheosis of what Walter Benjamin would call fascisization of art: in the aestheticization of the political in Godard's *Prenom Carmen*, as well as in his early works which were massively influential on Straub/Huillet. So there is no tension *between* sound and image, or within the various segments of music block for block in terms of meaning, such as the abstract "against" the supposedly concrete, the abstract "against" the representational. Thus no resistance is necessitated; a close-up of the singer is seen as a *necessary* close up of the *character* within the narrative. A false naturalization is given, the procedures of its being set up mystified. The point here is not that every procedure should be "there" on film, exposed or explained, as that is merely another level of documentation, "seeing what is 'really' taking place." The point is that the mystification of procedure, by making a coherent line of "rightness", harmony, quietude, end of struggle, about sound, image, and continuity, uninterrupted by the material, film, is the basic illusionist project.

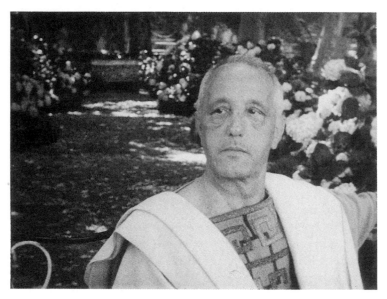

9 Jean-Marie Straub/Danielle Huillet, *History Lessons* (1974)

"All Straub/Huillet films, and Straub films (before their collaborative efforts) have, either as given (and seen as such) or as an unseen centre a persecuted character. (The persecuted outsider is never far from the central core of thought. The romantic male artist as outsider, communist, Jew, may be the figure of Jean-Marie Straub, though he is not an outsider, a communist, or a Jew.) This is the main reason for the impossibility of the films being able to produce themselves as material operations within a *social* space. They end up as personal stories or conventionalized images. As Straub quoted approvingly at one point, 'The symbol expands itself into an image' (Edinburgh Seminar, 1976), and, nearly ten years later, Huillet states, 'Landscapes, filmed as if they were characters,' to which Straub replies, 'Every landscape is a woman' (*Undercut* 7/8, 1983).

"*Introduction to the Accompaniment to a Cinematographic Scene by Arnold Schönberg* deals largely, inside its narrative, with Kandinsky's anti-Semitism. He invited Schönberg to the Bauhaus. He states, apparently categorically, though the letter does not survive, that 'for you it's not the same, you are an exception

[*Ausnahme*]. We make exceptions for great Jewish people like you.' The assumptions about what Kandinsky wrote are based on Schönberg's response stating, 'Because I have not yet said that for instance when I walk along the street and each person looks at me to see whether I'm a Jew or a Christian, I can't very well tell each of them that I'm the one that Kandinsky and some others make an exception of, although of course that man Hitler is not of their opinion' (4 May 1923, *Schönberg/Kandinsky, Letters, Pictures, Documents*, Faber & Faber, London 1984, p. 78). Straub/Huillet's interest is in this problem. The film takes, and asks the viewer to take, an emotional, i.e. unthought-out, stance against Kandinsky's assumed anti-Semitism. But we are against anti-Semitism. And against racism. And (here it gets more vague suddenly!) against sexism. And against. . . . This is a dealing in symptoms, causes remain un-explained. The material relations which produce, inside the Bauhaus, inside culturally sophisticated and philo-Semitic Berlin 'cultural circles' an overt anti-Semitism on the part of Kandinsky, this is not clarified at all. We are asked, in other words, to simply identify with the persecuted, an unthought, undistanciated, unreflexive identification. Brecht stated apropos another film, *Hangmen also Die*, 'It's against barbarism, but not the conditions which produce it!' Straub/Huillet in the *Schönberg* film do not deal with the conditions or relations either, let alone doing that *and* making a film which does work on film, on and against the codes, structures, forms, processes, positions, of filmic representation which *produce* and reproduce precisely the positions that they are 'against'. The identification mechanisms set up are those of bourgeois ahistorical cinema and theatre. Whatever disconnections do exist, such as allusions to the out-of-frame, actors' schematized placements, and so on, recuperate into a homogenous whole throughout. Stylistic variations from dominant cinema form, here, a stylistic totality for narrative completion. What is lacking is a complex interaction *between* filmic labour (presentation) and the internal event (representation)" (*Ark*, ibid.).

9 Fetishization of process

This concept has been alluded to and must be taken up further. The "unfolding of process" *per se* does not necessarily determine itself within a non-narrative film as different from a documentary representation, only it happens to be of process rather than plot. The example in relation to which this concept can be discussed is Mike Dunford's *Still Life with Pear*, (1973; prize at Knokke International Experimental Film Festival, Christmas 1974). First the filmmaker's description.

"A still life with a pear, lighted in a darkened space. The camera is focussed and after remaining in the first position for one minute is moved to right or left every thirty seconds according to a pre-recorded set of instructions. Centre section in which the pear is eaten. Third section in which the first instructions are repeated, but with the addition of a second person who eats the still life (pear), the camera uses the instructions as a basis of action, attempting to adapt them to the obstructive presence of the second person. A second sound-track is added to the first

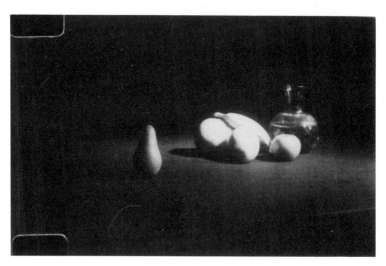

10 Mike Dunford, *Still Life with Pear* (1973)

in which the cameraman describes the *actual* actions that the camera makes.

"The film operates dialectically in that a prior structure was arrived at which denotes the operations to be performed by the camera and cameraman, and this, during the course of the film, interacts with the variables of the filming situation. A synthesis results which is a result of these two elements, and which was arrived at during the course of the film.

"The intention in this film was to deal with the act or intention to initiate a film, the prior structure for filming was limited to a simple time base, the distortion of this as a result of other factors renders the process as well as the elements involved perceptible" (Mike Dunford, "Filmmaker's notes," Knokke Festival, 1974, London Film Co-op Catalogue).

Dunford's notes are presented here as representative for the kind of notes the catalogue maintained, the kind of theorization that certain filmmakers attempted and were capable of, and also for the way in which filmmaking *before* 1974 seems to have been rooted in an unawareness of the instantiating of a documentariness which is, upon examination, the setting up of the pseudo-documentary. That is, the illusionist documentary wherein film, experimental or otherwise, poses as the adequate representation of an object or experience. Film becomes the window to life and, whether filmic process or love story, amounts formally to a parallel transparency. Had this not been seen as *the* theoretical problematic, it would have threatened to take the English experimental film into a retrogressive and ideologically reactionary position. The misreading of non-narrative cinema, a substitution into "unfolding of process," belies the existence of the film as procedure of transformational dialectic. Yet this film by Dunford was one of the most valuably important experimental films of the period precisely in its problematization of such issues, as the film itself raised these issues in the simultaneity of its "unfolding of visual process" against the continuum of sound "instructions" which only at moments synchronized. Also, Dunford's consistent autocritiques spoken and in program notes, as well as in his influential *After Image* essay,[6] and his attacks on the avant-garde from an engaged political position on the Left, served to force certain issues for the filmmakers at the London Filmmakers Co-operative. As much as did his formulations (around 1971/2) of structur*ing* as opposed to struct*ure*, in theoretico-political battle with the American model and with the London filmmakers' verbal back-sliding (which sometimes coincided with filmic advance).

One of Dunford's autocritiques follows: "Like many experimental avant-garde films, *Still Life with Pear* makes the technical practice of its production a part of the film. It seems to say, 'no distortion, everything exposed' but is a part of the distortion of empiricism and phenomenology, and ignores the role it has in social and political practice within bourgeois ideology. It is a good example of this reactionary form and fulfills its part in preventing questioning of the political nature of bourgeois perception, treating it as 'given', and hides the reality of the class struggle. It confines itself to the realm of aesthetics and exposure of its practices and necessitates the viewers' participation in these things. It fits very well into the 'non-political' area of the avant-garde. All perception of phenomena is unified by ideology and therefore political. *Still Life* is not non-political, it accepts the bourgeois class ideology of aesthetics, and the bourgeois idealist philosophy of empiricism, and necessitates participation in them. It does not confront them or its role in promulgating them, it supports the ideology of the propertied bourgeoisie and subverts the viewer into that ideology just as worker participation in factory management subverts the worker into capitalism. It was a product of my colonized consciousness and continues the process of colonization. I hope that nowadays you will criticize the film and ask the question 'whom does it serve and how?.' I no longer make such films" (Mike Dunford, *Arte Inglese Oggi 1960–1976*, Milan, November 1975). It must be noted that the polemic here had effects of making precise the possible political critiques from the Left, questions which an avant-garde that veered away from a materialist dialectic in film was begging. It is equally important to note that Dunford's current auto-critiques, and the theoretical positions they take up now, in the late 1980s, see the dangers of anti-modernist ultra-Leftism (not to mention ultra-Rightism of the post-modernists, endless apologists, via the simulacrum, of the status quo) to as extreme a degree as his critiques of bourgeois formalism did then. This makes work difficult, but there are few other possibilities.

After a gap of seven years, Dunford is again at work in experimental film and video, which he was one of the main filmmakers to formulate in the late 1960s, first with his beautiful, exemplary, minimalist 8 mm films in 1968, then at the London Filmmakers Co-op. Several of the films are concerned specifically with the determinations of the Co-op printer. The way things proceeded at the Co-op meant that various filmmakers consistently worked with others on their films, in teaching, for example, how the printer worked and of what practical and conceptual use it could be. The socialist structure of the Co-op preceded by a decade the intimations of film-collectivity in England, and was a model for it here and throughout Europe. The policy was instanced by Fred Drummond, Malcolm LeGrice, Mike Dunford, Annabel Nicholson, Gill Eatherley, Roger Hammond, Carla Liss, Barbara Ess, Simon Hartog, Steve Dwoskin, David Crosswaite, Lis Rhodes, and others.[7]

The fetishization of process, related to involvement with the 16 mm Co-op developing and printing equipment, became a major detour for some structural/materialist film, largely via the misappropriation of a materialist aesthetic to a positivist reading of the filmic apparatus. An ideology of process was evidenced as a fetishization of process finding its way into the profilmic (that which the camera is aimed at). Hence one can oppose, at an initial stage, this fetishization of work/process/technique to the concept of necessary labour, processing something into something *other*. *Process* must be brought back into the vocabulary minus it fetish meaning.

There is a further difficulty with *process*. Process was a term used by certain London filmmakers around 1966–9 with reference to one another's works and to the overall interests which they felt their films represented. But process can imply the process *of* an artist-subject, and this formulation was criticized in the early 1970s via an emphasis on the *material trace* and the notion of inscription. Filmic inscriptions would be produced as anonymous, would be in the film-process anonymized, rather than signifying an artist-subject both present-in-absence and always the imaginary referent of the text. Thus the material inscription of trace, the trace given not as some humanized effect, nor as some anthropomorphic cause, became a theoretically *concrete* construct for film-practice. The question as to the implication of an inferrable artist-subject also arose via apparatus-functions, such as hand-held camera movements, lighting, angle, distance, speed, and so on.

The question, for example, as to the determining of an unseen artist-as-subject-of-film via (in) camera-movement, was answered through the concept of *de-subjectivization*. This was seen as possible through repetitions and re-take, on the same or similar film-material (the distinctions between "same" and "similar" are taken up elsewhere.) It is thus a notion of a series of camera functions and editing functions which would de-subjectivize the resultant projected film-segment's procedure. This would then undermine, or negate, any ideal, or idealist, viewer's (ideal) subject-centre outside the film-trace's inscription. The project embarked upon through this critique was to make of the procedures a system wherein the viewer does not find him or her "self"; the gaze not trapped. This system would then disallow identification into procedure, in opposition (for example) to the way some abstract-expressionist and all neo-expressionist painting so often does not.

The same holds for music, writing, sculpture: expressionism, neo-or otherwise, inculcates the imaginary self-identifications that materialism radically struggles against through its (historical) dialectic, the latter in terms of both the spectator's sexual and economic objectivity and, not always separable, individual subjectivities.

The answer, though, tended towards a mechanistic materialism in some Co-op work, when the implications were not fully grasped; privileged status was given to the inscription *on* – in – the film-image (rectangle), thereby lionizing the trace (explicitly) and subscribing to crude distanciation and more problematically perceptual positivism (implicitly). Such distanciation and reliance on the *privileged place for the image*, deconstructed in time or not, was also inseparable from a reliance on meaning as given, however *motivated* against such a reliance it might have been. In such work the sexual signified solidified in capitalist patriarchy was merely "deconstructed" by the reproductions (a metaphysical intervention, thus) or through the mode or *style* of the reproduction's presentation (another metaphysic).

Deconstruction turned out to be juxtaposition, and "the *non*-denial of history," and "the *social* spaces of meaning," which

its adherents promulgated, turn out to be fixation upon metaphor. The overdetermination *by* social meaning of everything
else refuses materialist practice the possibilities of *producing
social meaning*. *Materialist process* disallows the indulgences of
setting up, figuring, an image, a sequence, and then somehow
"contradicting" it. What finally had to be learnt was that neither
the process, with the concomitant established subject-creator,
not the framed inscription of trace "out there" would suffice
for materialist practice. *Process* would have to be repossessed
for and in materialism. Which it then was. So would subject,
structure, perception, economy, sexuality, art. . . .

10 Deconstruction

Under the rubric of ego-psychology's death, there has evolved
a new sustaining of the subject. How? Through deconstruction.
There was a notion perpetuated by the editorial board of
Screen in the years 1973–83 that deconstruction could manage
via various film-strategies to avoid the traditional viewings'
ego-psychological identifications. The "mismatch" was the
most notorious of these ruses; film after film was analysed to
find a mismatch, or an assumed mismatch between ideology
and image (but the wrong way round!). John Ford's *Young Mr
Lincoln*, Dreyer's *Gertrude*, Lang's *The Cabinet of Dr Caligari*,
Welles' *Touch of Evil*, Hitchcock's *The Birds*, Berwick Street Collective's *The Nightcleaners*, Dwoskin's *Times For*, Godard/Gorin's
Tout Va Bien, all served this purpose; the effects were that then
a series of second generation cine-semiotic academics offered
the same positions on *their* good-object films: *Gilda, Waiting for
Mr Goodbar, Nashville, Dressed to Kill, Jeanne Dielman, Thriller*. Noel
Burch, who (in *Theory of Film Practice*) posited this theoretical
stance in the late 1960s and early 1970s in regard to Eisenstein's
Strike and *October*, as well as films by Lang, Dreyer, Antonioni,
and others, cannot be forgotten here; additionally, his position's
entrenchment was a detour from dealing with the possibilities
of a materialist, avant-garde, *experimental* film practice and its
necessary subversions.

"The fact that *The Cabinet of Dr Caligari* (1919), the first film to devolve fully and deliberately upon a deconstruction of the then barely instituted codes of transparence and the illusion of continuity, had to resort to the 'anti-codes' of theatrical expressionism . . . does not in any way detract from the radical nature of the break brought about by this film. The expressionist codes proved to have an infinitely more corrosive effect on those of the dominant forms of the cinema than they were able to have on those of the theatre to the extent that this film has almost always been expelled from cinema proper and classified under the heading of 'obsolete' theatricality, precisely perhaps because of the greater credibility that 'naturalist' and 'realist' projects have always enjoyed in the cinema as opposed to the theatre, where 'the willing suspension of disbelief' seems less univocal. . . . [Each of] the strategies . . . of *Dr Caligari* . . . [is] directed against a fundamental code of representation or narration in its contemporaneous stage of development" (Noel Burch, "Propositions," *After Image*, 5, 1974, p. 43). "This paridigmatic breakdown of codic operations makes *Caligari* the first self-reflexive filmic work, through which it largely escapes the ideological attitudes inherent in illusionist representation" (ibid., p. 44).

There follow a series of "do's" and "don't's" which ostensibly make for a deconstructive film, contesting this or that code (doors closing and not matching fully, eyelines looking the "wrong" way), or, alternately, suffusing all the shots of characters so as to use "the eye line match almost to the exclusion of any other type . . . doing away entirely with the pro-scenic frame of reference (the story)" (ibid., p. 44).

A hierarchical list of mechanically institutable functions within narrative which will result in deconstruction *of* narrative, apart from its voluntarist element, fails to take account of the spectator, or does so based upon crude assumptions of sociologistic truth, as if somehow such truths could be tested. If the wrong answers are given by a random sample, "false consciousness" is blamed. The problem with such a systematization is that it does not understand the dialectical nature of the world and its social relations, film included, though it utilized the terms for a quasi-moral substantiation of deconstruction. More importantly, it implicitly demands of film*making* the narrative basis, the screenplay with a story, the diegesis (the mental space of the film, as imaginable by the viewer) intact. What must be stressed is that for deconstructive cinema, the dominant apparati of production, distribution, and exhibition are maintained; only then can rules be obeyed for the proper questioning of codes!

The final problem with deconstruction, thus, is that questioning a code instantiates its normative power, repeating dominant power relations of representation, without acknowledging the repetition, and then subsuming it to a different *style*. Thus Dreyer "versus" Hitchcock, Welles "versus" Ophuls, Fellini "versus" Lang. What must be noted is Burch's equally vehement antagonism to those stylists who, according to him, mask conventional form through a heightened stylistic! Endless interpretation ensues, amongst academics, as to which filmmaker *really* does and which really does not deconstruct. The project as reactionary theoretical practice, politically and filmically, is never questioned.

11 Deconstruction and sexuality

Especially in those "deconstructive" films influenced by Godard and Straub/Huillet there is a ruse that the traditional patriarchal male subject is somehow avoided, submerged within the practice of the work. Yet these film "texts" have reaffirmed the central ideological male subject. For the epigones this was, through various mechanistically applied devices, meant to occur. A more acceptable "reconstruction" to follow. (In Britain such films were financed by the British Film Institute, 1976 to 1986.) A retrogressive decade of production thus in that part of the Independent Film Sector. They have thankfully been forgotten by history rather quickly.

A necessary lesson. At the level of *criticism*, a similar effect has been produced over the past decade, partially as a backlash against feminism, partly as the uninterrupted discourse of French criticism, which never acknowledged feminism as necessitating a battle against patriarchy and the sex-class men, male power, in the first place. Here Goethe's "the exception proves the rule" holds, for once. What was taken up was a vague "socialist feminism," that was also endorsed heartily by men who previously showed no signs of engagement with the politics of feminism, let alone any "interest in the subject". Socialist feminism "seems at every juncture to assume the term feminism can be dropped from the term socialist" (Christine Delphy, *Close to Home: A Materialist Analysis of Women's Oppression*, Hutchinson, London, 1984, University of Massachusetts Press, 1985, p. 140). In the decade's "radical" criticism, dominant representations of sexuality and "desire," and the bourgeois sexual conventions valorized by patriarchy, are incorporated and reproduced. A kind of representational libertarianism takes hold, in film and criticism, which reincorporates that which has been under attack from radical materialism. Deconstruction, as discussed, has its central place in the form and style of this end to struggle.

"The critique of deconstruction is right but no justification for a monolithic argument against all and every work engaging contemporary terms of representation and their production. Since film is never in itself *simply* radical, it is right and necessary to locate and critique the elements of its construction in ideological reproduction, but this is again no justification for a monolithic argument in which all films become indiscriminately and uniformly 'reactionary' and which avoids any consideration of the historical reality of the contradictions a film may represent *and decisively produce*" (Stephen Heath, "Narrative space," *Questions of Cinema*, Macmillan, London, and University of Indiana Press, 1981 and 1985).

"The historical reality of the contradictions a film may represent and decisively produce" includes, largely, sexist representations and the adaptation to this in academic rationalizing. This is a consequence of formulations which in the pristine argument against a monolithic stance, allow for "historical reality" to be "represented." Of course, contradictions are "found" when any film is spoken about, i.e. *afterwards*. Mainstream and recent so-called Independent Film, with its "historical subject-matter," does not produce contradictions-in-film. The contradictions occur because the social space in which such a film, *or anything*, exists is contradictory. Thus a film can be interpreted after the fact in relation to those contradictions, but they are not necessarily produced *by* the work. This is the sleight-of-hand of academic interpretive discourse, masking itself as weighty historical fact.[8]

Many such films, both in Britain and the United States, are "about" relationships, "about" a hero making existential decisions, about some Foucault-inspired correct "subject matter," "about" psychoanalysis (neither general and abstract, nor specifically concrete), "about" sociologico-personal "life," "about" sexuality and "desire," and so on. Many of the filmmakers, not coincidentally, are literary critics manqué, and vice versa (often two manqués residing in one body). Little trace of an art-practice of aesthetic production – *film*.

The critical position attending the mire is naive. Reference to one such: E. Ann Kaplan has written that certain fiction-films "might represent the start of a new language, a new Symbolic Law. Mothering seemed a fruitful area to explore. Mothering has been repressed in patriarchy but may, for that reason, provide a gap through which woman can begin to assert their voices and find a subjectivity" (E. Ann Kaplan, *Women and Film*, Methuen, London, 1983). Gap, Voices, Finding Subjectivity, Symbolic Law, all the *parts* for succumbing to the dilettantism French intellectuals are prone to. Late Kristeva/Barthes/Foucault/Derrida as soi-disant inspiration of all things! *Anything* can be written about by anyone (with *power*. And the powerless are powerless not to imitate this).

If anything has *not* been repressed in patriarchy, it is mothering (and the Law of the Symbolic). Mothering as constructed in patriarchy is not coincidentally the most oppressive, most conventional, position "for" women. It is defining via biologism a place *for* woman's "voice." This in the face of women, and feminism, having fought and fighting to eradicate that reduction to motherhood, and the reduction of women's voices to voice of mother. Kaplan assumes women have not been fighting for this, have no history. Otherwise how could she write of "beginning . . . to find a subjectivity in mothering" – with the help of film no less! Subjectivity is constructed in struggle, resistance, within and against the objective historical social–sexual positions given. Feminism, and specifically a materialist radical feminism, has taught that.

"Women will have to abstract themselves from the definition

'woman' which is imposed upon them. . . . Our fight aims to suppress men as a class, not through a genocidal, but a political, struggle. Once the class 'men' disappears, 'women' as a class will disappear as well, for there are no slaves without masters. Our first task it seems is to always thoroughly dissociate 'women' (the class within which we fight) and 'woman,' the myth. For 'woman' does not exist for us: it is only an imaginary formation, whilst 'women' is the production of a social relationship . . . which is based on the oppression of women by men, which produces the doctrine of the difference between the sexes to justify this oppression. What we believe to be a physical and direct perception is only a sophisticated and mythic construction, an 'imaginary formation' (Colette Guillaumin) which reinterprets physical features (in themselves as neutral as any others but marked by the social system) through the network of relationships through which they are perceived" (Monique Wittig, "One is not born a woman," *Questions Féministes*, no. 1, 1978; *Feminist Issues*, no. 1, 1981).

"To found a field of study on this belief in the inevitability of natural sex differences can only compound patriarchal logic and not subvert it: to pose woman as the specific object of oppression, we hide the fact that she is the object of oppression through the specific. Far from taking the Difference as the basis of our project, we should demolish it and denounce its falsity. Analysing how and why it must take on an ineluctable character: I must be a man or a woman; neither both nor something else . . . at the risk of getting lost. In this sense, building a solidarity indispensable to our survival may not rest on the elaboration of a feminine universe, on the idea of a shared nature of women. Which does *not* signify either that we are going to 'deny' our bodies, or 'want' to be men! The oppression of women is based on the appropriation of their bodies by patriarchy, on the restriction of sexuality within the framework imposed by the masculine–feminine opposition, the subjection of the woman in confinement to medical power, the contemptuousness of menstruation, the lack of recognition of sexuality. But recognizing this vast sexual oppression of women must not lead us to the conclusion that oppression derives from the body, or from sex; or that the body explains social opression. Woman's sex is denied, unrecognized. But that does not mean that woman's oppression derives from that lack of recognition. We must guard ourselves from a form of reflexive 'pan sexualism' which is only a coarse, disguised naturalism. If the category of sex has such an important position in patriarchal logic . . . it is because the social is able to make sexual forms seem obvious and thereby hide oppressive systems. . . . That is something that cannot be constructed in a problematic of the Difference. Nor in a prospective of the unutterable" (Monique Plaza, " 'Phallomorphic power' and the psychology of 'woman,' " *Questions Feministes*, no. 1, 1978, and *Ideology and Consciousness*, no. 4, Autumn 1978).

". . . the widespread theoretical schizophrenia of the Left on the subject of women's oppression. The contradictory analyses they produce are due to a desperate desire to continue to exempt men from responsibility for the oppression of women . . . men as the class which oppresses and exploits women. For a long time the socialist feminist current has represented within the Women's Liberation Movement an expression of a tendency to protect our enemies" (C. Delphy, "A materialist feminism is possible," *Close to Home*, op.cit.).

The above quotes are used to emphasize that the interrogation of these questions in a radically materialist way is important before "simply" utilizing concepts and "making an avant-garde independent film" or "critiqueing" one. The reproduction of dominant stereotypical forms of oppression is (unfortunately) justified by the concept of deconstruction, i.e. that in fact *any* political or sexual–political representation is problematic and deconstructable. In this way deconstruction functions as an alibi for *any* politics and polemic against representation. Its formalism, i.e. the imposition of deconstruction's style upon any text, at will, gives it an idealist motivation ignoring issues of the power of representation. Within the ideology of deconstruction, the positions taken in respect of (for example) "women" and "voice" matter not at all. Within a materialist film and critical practice, the reduction of women and "woman's voice" to mothering is out of the question. Out of the question both as to filmic and critical content. Equally out of the question any notion of a self-identified unitary viewer-position mystically in "knowledge," in filmic "truth" or "nature." The problematizing of the signifier, as it is called, is fundamental for film-political intervention and meaning-transformations. Interventions proceed into the processes of ideology: meaning, memory, "truth," "beauty," *power*.

With the concept and practice of deconstruction, the pleasure of the good object, i.e. the classical Hollywood narrative film, is maintained, whilst its liberal ideology imposes a "critique." Thus the academicism of the discourse is maintained, and resistance at the level of production, distribution, exhibition, and at the level of the male/female spectator, is annihilated. The analogy to cold-war liberalism is too close for comfort, but the analogy holds. And the greater degree of mystification which is co-present with these "counter-practices" means that, politically, illusionist practice is attempting to remain the norm. Through usages of "the norm," "sexual difference" functions as an alibi, keeping social relations intact. This is, for example, why recent academic texts ostensibly dealing with counter-cinema, and with cinematic practices against dominant narrative illusionism, end up with roughly 95 per cent analyses of Hollywood films and 5 per cent (almost invariably two or three examples) based on the odd experimental or avant-garde film. And of those it is those most amenable to narrative intepretation *even when ostensibly non-narrative* that receive analysis. The latter thus becomes the good conscience category of the producible pleasures of narrative illusionism, which creates the coherent ego and its pleasures, *and* allows *a posteriori* critique to take care of matters. Thus the viewing-lists of film courses, feminist, marxist, or simply "film appreciation," are remarkably similar, and virtually interchangeable. An equally reactionary alternative would be to "want the pleasures of voyeurism *simultaneous* with its critique . . . accessible movies, new identifications" (Kaplan, op.cit.).

12 Denial of semioticity

Against mainstream film semiology which valorizes "meanings" and "multiple meanings" for their own sake, called "polysemic discourses," Annette Kuhn has written on the radical import of semioticity-denying possibilities in avant-garde film. Such positions are as rare as they are useful: ". . . the opposition between movement and stasis is realized in the relentless return to photographs as objects of representation and the constant and apparently random movement of the camera over these objects. The possibility of contemplation offered by photographs is recouped and even radically undercut by the continually moving picture. At those moments in the film when meaning does seem about to emerge – when the camera zooms back to offer a larger and more unified perspective – the solution to the riddle of the profilmic space is immediately displaced by the denial of such space implied in the revelation that the film image is not 'reality' reproduced, but another image reproduced. This posing of a puzzle and refusal of a solution provides a recurring structure for the film, and a repeated denial of the spectator's efforts to impose meaning.

"The repeated denial of meaning . . . is effectively an assertion of meaninglessness, a project of radical asceticized deconstruction.[9] (Use of this term by Kuhn is oppositional to that previously discussed.) Such a deconstruction is effected by a virtually complete refusal of cinematic codes: *not only codes of the dominant cinema, but also the codicity of the structural film itself.* In this film the illusory three-dimensional space of dominant cinema is only referred to in the moment of its displacement by the flat perspective of what is represented – still photos. The constant zooming, precisely because in this instance it cannot alter its perspective, serves to emphasize the very lack of depth in the image. The suppression of meaning production as a cinematic process is a *structuring* feature of the film in its constant movement into and out of focus, and in the graininess and undifferentiated colour of the image, all of which constitute references to the material character of the image-producing technology – here, filmstock and the optics of the camera lens. This is associated with a refusal of the illusion of homogenous filmic space, not only in the sense already suggested, but also by the collapsing of on-screen/off-screen space evident in the movement between the edges of the filmed image – coterminous with the screen – and the edges of the photographs, so that the space of the film is subject to a process of constant redefinition. The repetitions, the radical refusal of semioticity, the unfixed nature of the space articulated by the film, all serve to operate against the kind of closure associated with a defined and homogenous film space" (Annette Kuhn, "Notes for a perspective on avant garde film," Hayward Gallery, London, 1977). The theoretical positions elucidated by Kuhn here obviate the individual importance of a specific film being discussed. As experimental film-practice can pre-empt narrative analysis through denial of semioticity, a point made by Kuhn – the effacement through the process of the film, through the production process itself – a different kind of semiotics will be necessary. The problematic becomes one of locating that new semioticity.

The denial of semioticity which Kuhn stresses must be related to the concept of the non-naturalness of all social formations. Since everything is constructed, no "nature" pre-existent, the production process of a film, and the production of its meanings, can be recognized as arbitrary. It is arbitrary inasmuch as it is each time an ideological position rather than the representation of a prior essence, truth, or nature. It is in that sense that the concept of the arbitrary must be seen as inseparable from the concept of meaninglessness. Meaning does not inhere, it is formed, produced by complex processes, within film and without. On that level the division between art and life must be seen not as life being art, aestheticizing life in other words, but rather as art being life, in the sense that all discourses are inseparable from history and the real. Film is a cultural discourse, both material and ideological. To be more specific, the ideological is also material, the material of ideology. Material must not mean just that which you can touch, some object.

It is with these attempts at definition in mind that Realism must be redefined. Realism of another kind. Brecht's "a realism not defined formally" means not sticking to the *forms* that Realism has been cemented to in the past. But we cannot take Brecht as an orthodox guide, as he spoke equally often of "representing reality, the way it is" (*die Realität widergeben*) as of "Realist, that means consciously influenced by reality," another matter entirely (Bertolt Brecht, "Über den Realismus," Suhrkamp Verlag *Gesammelte Werke*, vol. 16, 1938–40).

The implications of this argument are specific. Certain

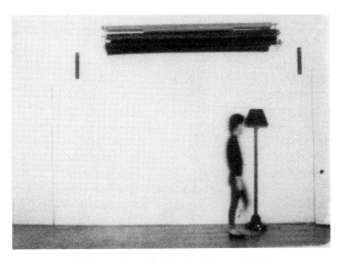

11 Lucy Panteli, *Motion Picture* (1981)

signifiers cannot be radically undercut. The image of a pregnant woman, so the argument already went in 1969 around the Filmmakers Co-op, is locked into a signification system so ideologically overdetermined that no other kind of operation affecting the editing, zooming, focusing, camerawork, subject-position, in the audience, off-screen space, or sound, can "subvert" it. It remains culturally enclosed and politically solidified in meaning. Yet its obverse, the lack of a potent signifier, the filmic creation of meaninglessness, can never be of a *pure* or *final* meaninglessness. That would be a transcendental trap. All signifiers exist in history and in time. Obviously, a space is not a sixteenth-century space if it is a twentieth-century space, even if the latter cannot be chronologically or perceptually fixed or held as "room," just (referential) elements in space which one (without success) attempts to construct into a coherent imaginary space. Class is signified by certain referents, certain film reproductions. But if they are not "arrested" (Gidal) or "held into a representation" (Heath), if they do not allow the fixing and closing of imaginary space, time, narrative, then there is a constant conflict between the attempt to see, to make a scene, to imagine a time and place, and the simultaneous impossibility, the endless meaninglessness of all signifiers, any

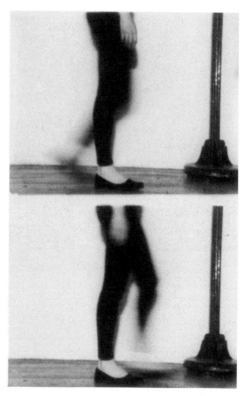

12 Lucy Panteli, *Motion Picture* (1981)

meaning-construction thereby presented as construction, as production-process. The politics of such cinema is the politics of that. A denial of the process and function of problematizing significatory objects in film leads to an abstract, formal practice that is *not* linked to questions of representation. Thereby we would be left simply with a suppression and repression of the problematics of meaning in cinema. But "abstract" and "form" must be terms not held to such definition. The dominant position for the viewer, consuming seamless narrativity and its voyeurist "pleasures," can be opposed by abstract work in/through/against form.

". . . to make different films differently. This is necessary partly because, as Althusser pointed out, 'It is the intermediation of the ruling ideology that ensures a sometimes teeth-gritting "harmony" between the repressive state apparatus (police, courts, prison, army) and the Ideological State Apparatus (religion, school, family, parties, culture, press), and between the different Ideological State Apparatuses'. We can make that teeth-gritting visible. Look and listen, such films would say, this is a construction constrained by the materiality of the signified *and* the signifier, and this is something like the way social reality is also constructed, but we are showing that both unitary complete social individuals (subjects) and units of social reality (facts) – conflated as subjects of filmic discourses – are multiple, that reality is a multiple and differential series" (Phillip Corrigan, "(Re)making it new, independence and film form," *Undercut*, no. 1, March 1981, pp. 19–21).

"This state of affairs – the result of a history which inscribes woman as subordinate – is not simply to be overturned by a contemporary practice that is more aware, more self-conscious. The impasse confronting feminist filmmakers today is linked to the force of a certain theoretical discourse which denies the neutrality of the cinematic apparatus itself. A machine for the production of images and sounds, the cinema generates and guarantees pleasure by a corroboration of the spectator's identity. Because that identity is bound up with that of the voyeur and the fetishist, because it requires for its support the attributes of the "non-castrated," the potential for illusory mastery of the signifier, it is not accessible to the female spectator who, in buying her ticket, must deny her sex. There are no images either *for* her or *of* her" (Mary Ann Doane, "Woman's stake: filming the female body," *October*, no. 17, 1981, pp. 23–4).

In terms of the feminist struggle, though a man cannot "be" a feminist, the refusal has been to allow images of women (or men) into my films (with two or three aberrations – indulgences produced for consumption in a state of self-identificatory narcissism. Rather than respond "why not," why not say why?), since I do not see how those images can be separated from the dominant meanings. The ultra-left aspect of this may be nihilistic as well, which may be a critique of my position because it does not see much hope for representations for women, but I do not see how, to take the main example given around 1969 before any knowledge on my part of, say,

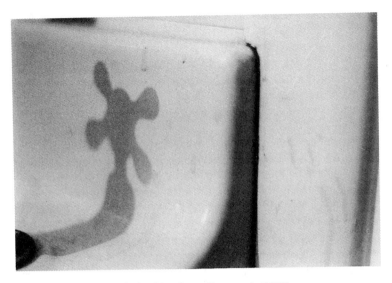

13 Nicky Hamlyn, *Guesswork* (1979)

semiotics, there is any possibility of using the image of a naked woman, or a pregnant woman – at that time I did not have it clarified to the point of any image of a woman – other than in an absolutely sexist and politically repressive patriarchal way at this conjuncture. And no images of men because they are as overdetermining and overdetermined.

"This is the extreme formulation of a project which can define itself only in terms of negativity. If the female body is not necessarily always excluded within this problematic, it must always be placed within quotation marks. *For it is precisely the massive reading, writing, filming of the female body which constructs and maintains a hierarchy along the lines of a sexual difference assumed as natural.* The ideological complicity of the concept of the natural dictates the impossibility of a nostalgic return to an unwritten (i.e. natural) body" (Doane, op.cit.).

Thus the answer is not, simply, to have the female body positioned differently, as would be the example of the represented woman simply "looking back" at the viewer and audience, whether male or female. As Stephen Heath has written: "A recent article on 'The avant garde and its imaginary' was ended by its author, Constance Penley, as follows (in *Camera*

Obscura, no. 2): 'If filmic practice, like the fetishistic ritual, is an inscription of the look on the body of the mother, we must now begin to consider the possibilities and consequences of the mother returning the look.' To which Peter Gidal whose writings had been a major focus of discussion replied: 'The last words of your piece say it all. You search for the simple inversion, the *mother looking back*. I consider the possibilities of the not-mother, not-father, looking or not.' "

Heath continues, "The exchange seems to crystallize much of what is most importantly at stake. To invert, the mother returning the look, is not radically to transform, is to return as well the same economy, the same dialectic of phallic castration, the same imaginary (and cinema in the fiction film has always and exactly been concerned to consider the possibilities and consequences within the fetishistic ritual, including the constitutive threat of its endangerment, the play of eye and look, vision and lack); the difference inverted is also the difference maintained" (Stephen Heath, "Difference," *Screen*, Autumn 1978, pp. 97–8).

Additionally, the argument has to be made that denial and negativity as previously discussed by Doane has been misused in film theory, which has avoided the fact that all theory is polemics. New thought comes from struggle, and all polemics are based on "negative" resistance to and radicalization against existing power.

13 Andy Warhol's *Kitchen* (1965)

Kitchen is a production of a problematic sexuality in the viewer. It is a forerunner of structural/materialist film. It is a "classic" of the avant-garde, largely *unseen*. *Kitchen* is in black and white, of sixty minutes' duration. "A murder is committed on the table in a white kitchen. A photographer keeps coming into the frame; the actors interrupt what they are doing and pose for pictures; pages of script are handed to the actors, who follow them. The happenings inside and outside of the frame are equally important to the interchange. Everyone sneezes throughout the

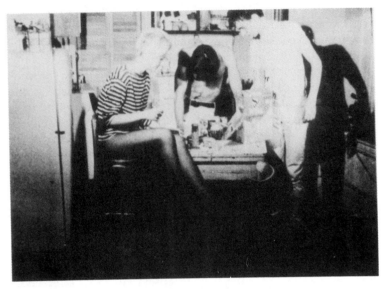

14 Andy Warhol, *Kitchen* (1965)

film" (Jonas Mekas, "Filmography of Andy Warhol," in John Coplan's *Andy Warhol*, New York Graphic Society, 1971).

In *Kitchen* sexed positioning by the actors is always an enactment, taking account of the camera to whom it is addressed. The enactment equally takes account of *film* as such. Film in Warhol's usage is unceasing, makes demands *as film*, aggresses by its refusal to abstain: the camera keeps running. In Warhol's work, often, and in this case in particular, the film is made up of thirty-minute takes, that is, thirty minutes of uninterrupted filming. Sexual role-playing within the script is imbricated with the constant persistence of the cinematic apparatus, the machine, at work.

JO [played by Edie Sedgewick]: Joe's coming up in the world.
JOE: My coffee's coming up.
MICKEY: My left knee's coming up this time. I don't know why you go in for it, it's not your type really.
JOE: Well, I can go down for a time. That Mexican – let me tell you about this fabulous Mexican I met.
MICKEY: No more, thank you.

JOE: He was all in white and very concerned, just like he'd just got thrown out of a pajama party or something. And speaking of pajama parties, where's my coffee?
JO: Joe darling, I don't believe a word you're saying.
JOE: That's always where my troubles are. I just don't have the time to be believed by everyone.

And so on. The script, by Ronald Tavel, is adhered to whenever the actors can remember the lines, which is most of the time. When they forget, they chatter, down to silence. To help them "remember" (and even remembering is enacted, "quoted") there are copies of the script on the table in the kitchen. There is a copy under the calender on the wall which one actor in particular keeps looking at. But there is no evidence when "picking up a phrase" that it is from the "script." The script itself becomes a pre-text.

The film plays constantly on the actors' awareness of the camera, of seeing and being seen. Edie constantly poses self-consciously, acts her part with sudden changes of mood. We are to assume these changes are called for in the scenario, but the changes become so *sudden* as to produce the effect on the viewer of acts being "quoted," being in themselves imitations of instructions, mechanistically employed. This produces the startling effect on the viewer. The dialectic engaged in is constantly on this plane. When Edie moves her enactments into high camp, sneezing two or three times per sentence, broadening her speech and extending her vowel-sounds in mock heroics, there is no evidence that the switch "back" to another style of speech and gesture is any more "real." The part is played to perfection in unerring ambivalence of naiveté/ sophistry. Identity is not established; attempted identifications split into (the viewer's) *un*knowing.

EDIE: Who were you with in the shower, Jo? Joe!
JOE: Who cares, you don't have sex with a name.

This sentence mimics within the narrative the process that is produced *by* the film. Namely, the positioning of the viewer as asexual, which is, and can be put to, social use. Such asexuality's radicalism is the effect of a lack of identity in the sexual role. Thus asexuality must stress its constant conflict with the subjective and objective histories of the viewer-as-subject. Then it is *not* a matter of some unfounded (viewer-as-) subject, somehow simply neither male nor female. The viewer is posited neither in "difference," as male versus the female spectacle, nor as female persona against the exigencies of dominant patriarchal content and form. Instead, difference is elided, enlarging the differentiation of sexualities *rather than* predetermined (heterosexual) positions of male and female occasionally "varied" always in respect to the norm. What is attempted is the production of a sameness through the elision of the oppressions of difference. Yet this in no way means the suppression of different histories for men and women – precisely the conflict of those histories with the attempted radical break is what could produce a next step.

Little is left, with *Kitchen*, when the process is ended, when the film is over. It might do to recall that in most cinema much is left, as most of the meaning is left, and extracted only after the process has been concluded, i.e. after the film is over. Meanings, and their retained values, are surplus values in meaning. These have been expropriated from the work-process of film-viewing and the individual–social process of meaning-making. This raises the political question in aesthetics which must be answered: in whose or what interests is this exploitation for consumption of meaning? Opposed to this is the concept of production, a discourse, not a religious moment or concept separate from actual *use*. The viewer as imbricated with his/her sexualities in the possible uses to which these are put, becomes relevant politically in such a cinematic theory of useful, transformative function.[10] The lack of expropriated surplus value of extractable meaning in *Kitchen*, the fact that so little remains, means it has been used, must have been used in-process, during the viewing, during the film-as-duration. This could equally leave meanings as use*less*, or not. But when useless, then at least not under the illusion of usefulness.

Here is the point at which so-called nihilism can be materialist and productive: when it is opposing uselessness not to usefulness, but to the illusion of usefulness.

The emptying-out of potent signifiers, of meaning, the cinematic "little is left" is a materialist engagement with the production process. Here the material is used up, processed, rather than somehow retaining a fetish existence which has to be maintained for constantly repeated consumption. *Kitchen* is thus opposed to dominant cinema's operations. The viewer's imbrication, as opposed to endless interpretation *of,* means she/he is in a different political position. The specificity of that kind of difference must then be analysed for each particular work.

I will not discuss here the more overt parodying of sexual role, in *Kitchen,* and the equation of impotence with male sexuality, obsessive repetition in compulsive speech and gestural act with the active female sexuality. Both are parodies of existing conventionalized forms without an interior logic to sustain the characterizations as they appear. The diegesis, i.e. the interior imaginary narrative, is not given as a logic of character, action, or any "true." There are no *a prioris.*

Lacan's "constant rememoration" becomes a memory-less carrying-on, endless attempt at memory as to what one's sexual identity is, or was, or could be, or could have been. Each new position taken in the actor's attempt to "act male" or "act female" immediately brings with it the closures of the respective convention, and those closures impel the role to new imaginative (i.e. *imagination* in Coleridge's usage, as necessitating *thought*) attempts to rid the self of the claustro-phobia of specific sexual identity. This endless process, this memory-less carrying on in endless rememoration attempt, is thus a dialectical and conflict-ridden process, because as one attempts to gain an identity the closures of its conventions impel attempts at change and transformation, at the same time as one is attempting memory and the hold of a previous identity that may have been "right" or "good" or "satisfactory." Sexual dialectics on this level continue through the film. The oppressions awaiting each position therefore motor the next. The real as residue, where nothing else is left, no "choices," is the material of such politics.

What is constantly undermined through *Kitchen's* filmic speech and gestural procedure is recourse to metaphor. The fictions metaphor imposes are disabled by the described *process;* for metaphor to function it must properly hold.

If that hold is simultaneously broken, if meaning is produced through opposition and conflict, then metaphor's transcendental, mythic, timeless necessities for stability cannot obtain. Once metaphor operates, its meanings adhere to whatever object they are formed through and with. A materialist process disallows this. In addition, it disallows the retrogression that occurs in aesthetic production whenever metaphor is given currency.

During certain viewings (such as of *Kitchen*) you find yourself placed with difficulty. The position of unknowing can be through film, or camera, operations whose aesthetic systematizations over time are not made recognizable and "known." A materialist film makes the viewer a not-knower. In the position of not-knower, one as viewer is forced to take up ideological positions, *as ideological*, political positions *as politics*, aesthetico-ideological politics as that. Herein eradicated is the possibility of consuming passively through emotion, nostalgia, good conscience, and so on. The illusion of something being given is not given.

Thus, through a materialist film process a female viewer cannot be placed as paternal knower against her own interests, against real subjective and objective histories of struggle. Equally impossible is the making of a victim, against her sex-class interests, via the route of "pleasure" and "desire." Political struggle in representation is not about what I or you know or don't know, but about demands and resistance. Thus, a film which gives no narrative completion and no implied fictive truth to that which is represented functions differently from one that does. *Kitchen* begins certain operations which could be developed into materialist cinema, and for which it could be useful. It itself still makes sure that the viewer is recouped by the representation through character, anecdote, coherent imaginary on-and-off-screen space, synchronized sound not in conflict with the anthropomorphic. Yet one is viewing it without *an* end, neither a narrative which can be followed nor an implied narrative which can be phantasmed ahead and then retroactively justified, literally or technologically. Without end, too, the moment to moment movement of it, always in reference to the moment to moment movement of you, as problematic. Thus the viewer as separated, precisely not co-opted into a mythical oneness of you and the representational process.

The nihilism alluded to previously connects to the movement towards stasis, the static camera position refusing to become a mobile anthropomorphic "eye." The constant running out and down, towards entropy (when the film reel runs out/when the motor stops), unpleasure principle and death-drive. Possibly this persistence of movement (camera, light, grain, time) upon that which moves less (the represented action) makes this nihilistic stance. The machine (camera, projector) as unstoppable, durable and unendurable.

The emphasis on materiality should not permit the assumption that for the viewer such film is "unrepressed," or that the viewer, in a state of unrepression, responds to what is materially indisputable. As if materialist meaning were a matter of lifting a veil, betraying truth (or worse, ever-present truth!) beneath. The point to make is the opposite: that a materialist process operates in contradiction and through conflict with the repressions of social sound and vision in the viewer viewing. What is materially present is that each moment of sound, and image, has concrete effects which incorporate, and are incorporated by, the viewer in his/her specificity. This cannot exclude unconscious desires, phantasies, projections, assumptions, needs, and so on. The viewer in that sense becomes a specific effect of a view*ing*, and the materialist problematic is located there. The material relations which form the "I" include aesthetic production. Yet the I's collectivities have their social effects. In such a conceptualization, there can be no real material "present," as the signifier signifies each moment something not-there. That other place is a social space of represented (or unrepresentable) social, sexual, economic relations, or/and a place of the unconscious.

The unconscious may be *less* than the significations of "lived" desires, not more. The ucs not as excess, spilling over. The ucs as always less, the splitting of identity-constructions caused by *that* lack, nothing "there" to substantiate a structure of self into fictions of "more." The ucs has its own histories. It('s less) is at odds with the more conscious life. Wherefrom repetitions to reify against that less, leading to nothing but the fetish of identity.

If the observer is part of the system observed (Wittgenstein, *Tractatus*) no objects or forms can precede perceptual activity.

Yet they do. An example is acetate's recording of light, producing images and sounds (sound-tracks are optical). Often, in early Warhol work, the recorded light produces a seeming stasis via a reduction of depth of the image, due to the harsh lighting's effect of flattening out. The image lasts for half an hour per roll of 1200 feet of film in *Kitchen*. The image is made up of hard light/dark contrast, allowing space to be constituted only through action. Thus movement breaks the flatness of the black/white space represented. The flat, stark contrasts of shape become spatially constituted in depth, with volume, and so on, only when someone or something moves or is moved. At the same time, ideology "resides in" all representations, and the viewer is embedded in the ideological; film's primary materialist function can hardly be ascribed to the (conscious or unconscious) viewer-as-subject. There is a material-real, namely the film (see p. 127 on "the real").

The self is a cipher, an effect of the apparatus' ineffable stare, stare-as-duration. This cipher, this "I," is always placed contradictorily, but depending on the material bases (the film and the viewer's historical, economic, sexual relations), such contradictory positioning can lead but equally can not lead to opposition. The repressed social ideologies of the individual guarantee that dialectical conflict does not insure a "progressive" position. Self as cipher, effect of, and within, material relations of cinematicity means such film practice can be an act of negation. It produces conflictual effects, effects *against*. The alternative to a practice of negation is a difference-constituting practice which fetishizes "difference," a range of acceptable stimuli, via one stylistic or another, leading to the idealist oppressions of an "open" or "free" text. The latter persist against the processes and problematics of Negation, Politics, Practice, Theory, *Film*.

In *Kitchen* the actor's roles are constantly taken up and let go at will, at whim. Any "one" characterization, or "person," is inseparable from characterizations which disallow belief in the actor's reality *and* in the assumed character-role. The unfixed locus of the actor's presenting of self, the lack of a support structure for the aura of the image, is, in Warhol's early films, fragile and constantly resituated, a series of poses all given as a series of poses, none of which could be dislocated from a *real* underneath. Thus, an anti-psychological notion of character is enforced. Roles and masks are never metaphysically united in a body, spirit or essence are not found to reside anywhere at all. The residue of all this is a different film-material history. It is as if such work were the process of a culture which no longer necessarily reproduces the bourgeois. Thus the work is in advance of the present.

Such work remains unseen, elided, as the contradictions increase, and their author's social position increasingly has a different objective and meaning. "Andy Warhol" is not the work, is of no interest to the work, though simultaneously the work is more and more covered by the social meanings the persona makes as a context (Warhol's death didn't obliterate this).

"Warhol was a key figure in the development of the American avant-garde film, but appears too late to have any such impact, around 1966–8, in England. The innovations in the late Warhol movies, *Lonesome Cowboys* (1968), *My Hustler* (1965), and *Bikeboy* (1967) that most appeal to English filmmakers are his use of the so-called strobe cut ('as an alienation device,' we wrote at the time) whose flash frames and blips were caused by in-camera editing during synchronized sound shooting, and his denial of the space–time continuum, within a single, extended (frequently thirty-five minute) take. Interesting though these innovations were, they were all distinctly outside of technical financial possibility for most filmmakers in England at that time. There were concerns here with formal innovations such as straying focus and zoom, arbitrary pans and the mismatch of camera and projection speeds. To the extent that these concerns were transmitted to English filmmakers, they were transmitted as already codified" (David Curtis, "English avant-garde film: an early chronology," *Studio International*, Film Issue, November 1975, pp. 176–82).

Feeling like a voyeur watching Warhol's *Couch* (1964, silent) is precisely not to be in the position of a voyeur. "A nude woman on a couch tries to get a man's attention. Later there is much banana-eating, and love-making attempts are seen, man to man, as other men sit in front of the couch, or walk around it. The camera is stationary, framing the couch" (Mekas, op.cit. p. 148). The film is made up of single takes lasting two and three-quarter minutes each. Each tableau lasts for one such 100-foot reel's length, then the next. There is no automatic linkage between one and the next, except that upon occasion one person from one shot will appear in another, with no narrative relation to the foregoing appearance. Often people look straight into the camera, then get on with their "business," in and out of frame. Movement is directed as much at the frame edges as within the frame, though the camera-frame does not move; by remaining static, its ineluctableness persists. The machine *cinema* foregrounds itself, as endless and impossible record, without teleology. The systemic structure does not allow for any narrative crests and waves; those that the viewer positions him/herself in relation to and through are of his/her making, as there is no superior or anterior purpose that can be somehow adequately divined or inferred. Each sequence is simply preceded by, and followed by, another of equal length, with another event or series of events, with different, sometimes the same, people, acting different, sometimes the same, roles.

The London Filmmakers Co-op catalogue (1972) described the film this way at one point (regrettably my notes): "The most important of Warhol's early works. A nude woman on a couch tries to get a man's attention. The woman, Kate Heliczer, sucks Rufus' nipples. Gerard Malanga sucks Kate's cunt and asshole. Softcore love, sex avec le couch, et cetera. Later there's much banana eating, and lovemaking attempts man with man, and vice versa (?). Other men sit around, walk around, in and out of frame. The camera is stationary, framing the couch. The girl with enormous tits tries (vainly) to seduce a motorbike polisher, sweet-sweet nothing boy. People just sit around. Looking at one another. Looking at the camera, at Andy, at nowhere et cetera. Stillness. Movement as habit, as recurrence. No goals. Just there. (Et cetera). With Gerard Malanga, Piero Heliczer, Naomi Levine, Gregory Corso, Allen Ginsberg, John Palmer, Baby Jane Holzer, Ondine, Kerouac, and others, some dead, some alive."

14 The stare and voyeurism

It is the stare here that works towards countering the identificatory process, by presenting the stare's presence. Self-conscious
viewing can be instigated this way, as it similarly can be by
the reflexivizing of the constant attempt to arrest an image.
Making the mechanism apparent (stare, arrestation attempt,
etc.) *whilst* it is in operation is a constituent part of countering
identificatory processes. Posited within such formulations of,
for example, the stare in Warhol, is a self situated in its
self-alienation. That is the place from which the stare is sited,
no humanized self finally left. View*er* becomes (a) view*ing*.
Without stabile self, totalized identificatory projections and
introjections can be barred; a first step. The anti-illusionist
project foregrounds mechanisms of cinema in the viewing,
denying possibilities of an imaginary oneness of viewer and
viewed. Seemingly endless duration produces itself *as* duration,
across the continuum of the stare. For this "continuum" to
appear seamless, as conventional narrative films demand, it
needs endlessly *interrupted* duration, edited for the illusion of
a continuum. The very opposite of time-as-duration. Yet the
processes engaged against identification cannot operate in a
vacuum, to somehow "make" a *non*-illusionist final work; rather,
an anti-illusionist project is *attempted*.

The question of voyeurism has to do with the *power*, or
imaginary power, of the viewer in the imaginary scene projected on-screen. It is the denial of apartness that motivates
voyeurism, the illusion of partaking, and for this illusion
to function, identification with the other must take place.
Whether it has to do with sympathetic feelings or sadistic ones
is structurally immaterial. It is in the face of powerlessness to
be other than the ineluctable, isolate self that identifications of
voyeurism originate.

"I saw a film recently by Oshima. It was called *Death
by Hanging*. This person who was hanged doesn't die and
comes back and talks.. He was accused of raping a woman
who was riding a bicycle and he had already had a phantasy
about raping a woman riding a bicycle. In the phantasy, this

woman was coming from the right into his vision, and he saw her and raped her. But when he actually raped a woman, she was coming from the left. And he couldn't do it until he put himself into another position so that she was coming from the same side as in the phantasy. It somehow reminds me of just the discrepancy between the expected and the mystery" (speaker in audience, "Discussion with Peter Gidal," *Millennium Film Journal*, vol. 1, no. 2, 1978).

Identification, and being put into that position of needing coherence, male spectator and perpetrator of the rape, relies heavily on a kind of patriarchal eroticization, which all cinema spectacle – all spectacle – is. And that eroticization is one which cannot be completely dissociated from concepts such as rape. This explains the connection between the voyeuristic positioning and the secure viewing of a narrative completion. Freud mentions that men have this amazing capacity to not think of anything other than completion and fulfillment – fulfillment in a very teleological sense, sexually and otherwise. Lou-Andreas Salome contrasts culturally produced female practicality against Freud's assumptions of "female impracticality," and against culturally produced male teleologies. "Fulfillment" through power-*over*, i.e. rape. So one can neither separate the viewing of a spectacle in a dark room from voyeurism, nor separate that from the rape analogy in the above quote.

"I felt horrified by the film *The Entity*. I came out of it shaking, I'm still trying to get over it. . . . I cried for quite a lot of the film. I've been in the campaign [Women against Violence against Women] for two years and I've seen a lot of pornography and a lot of violence against women, but this film is different, this film is aimed at the ordinary woman. I am an ordinary woman, and I was shaken, hurt, by the continual scenes of a woman raped – I'm still hurt by it. That film capitalizes on and exploits women's pain and women's fear. There were very few women watching it, it was generally men, the women there whom we talked to were like ourselves, they were shaking and very, very frightened, and angry. This film's going out on general release, it's being sold as general entertainment. A lot of women will be going to see it not knowing what it is. I hope the picket will warn women so they know what it's about."

FEMALE INTERVIEWER (from LBC Radio, London): "It's one of the occasions when I've come out of the cinema feeling frightened of the men who were coming out of the cinema with me."

"Yes, I kept my eyes towards the women, I knew my reaction to the men would be very angry, what I'd see in them. The writers and makers of the film want men not to be seen as responsible for rape – instead it's this thing called the entity – this feeds the male myth and male phantasy, the male lie about rape, that women want it, that women ask for it, that men have no responsibility for it . . . it's such a horrendous film in that it's so realistic. They have a strong, independent woman who has stepped out of line, and her punishment for stepping out of line is rape. This is the way men have treated women, do treat women, this is not 'just' a piece of cinema. We address ourselves as feminists to women, women who are feeling victimized, it's those we talk to. . . ."

FEMALE INTERVIEWER: "Is there any evidence that films do any real harm?"

"If women come out of the cinema feeling victimized then that is harm – you can't measure the norm. Men feel their own power enhanced. That's the norm. You can't measure it. I say if one woman, one single solitary woman felt bad about that film, that is harm, that is sufficient reason for us all to be angry.

FEMALE INTERVIEWER: "What further action are you taking besides picketing this evening?"

"That's up to the mass of women. We have a right to be furious that men can make a film for their pleasure that is based on women's rightful fear" (Rachel and Sarah, surnames not given, from Women against Violence against Women, LBC Radio, London, Interview, 8.15 p.m. 30 September 1982).

Later on in the same program, Harold Schneider, the film's maker, is interviewed, and he states: "There's only been a small percentage of negative reaction in the previews we've organized so far. I don't know why you feel the way you do. We did a lot of studies prior to making the film."

FEMALE INTERVIEWER: "It seems you decided to make a film that makes money: sex makes money, and the supernatural is making money, so let's put the two together."

SCHNEIDER: "It could be seen that way, but that would be wrong" (ibid).

Which fits neatly with Julia Kristeva's: "I would say that everything has to be shown, and then, afterwards, things can be critically discussed. I believe a work of art produces sensations, and thereby for the reader/viewer the artwork takes care of those problems, so that they take place in the imagination, and therefore do not become dangerous. It becomes a true purging." She continues, equating feminism with Nazism, and Marxism with anti-Semitism, concluding: "Farewell to politics . . . feminism included, that last of the power-seeking ideologies" (Peter Gidal, "On Julia Kristeva", *Undercut*, no. 11, February 1984, pp. 14–20).

Positing a different viewer, countenancing the voyeurism and rape analogies, must take account of the fact that there is no film which subverts the real in an empirically immediate way; the real "resists," forcing struggle. Equally, there is no one film which somehow changes the viewer in a kind of positivistic subjectivist manner. An obsessive in life is not criticized necessarily by the image of a non-obsessive in a film! The woman in Hitchcock's *Marnie* is not the same as a women in her room. "Why does Vera Myles go into the cellar after what happened upstairs, in *Psycho?*" "Because that's what women do, in films" ("Alfred Hitchcock interview," *The Times*, November 1983). That which *is*, the material real, is only subvertable by another material real, not by an image *of* a material real. Simultaneously each material *real* is a semiotic, is a meaning, is an image *of*. Yet an image is no less a material real, which can be subverted by another image, another material real. This means that the problematizing of representation, meaning, meaninglessness, etc., can be produced *in-film*, filmically, but that the social real, the extra-cinematic, is not contingent or cathartically at one with it. Otherwise one would be solidifying the notion, yet again, of film proffering a "higher" individual via vicarious activity or, more perversely, a viewer feeling so good about feeling bad, the standard liberal response to politics viewed, from "documentaries" about starvation to *The Nightcleaners*, (See Claire Johnston and Paul Willemen, "The Nightcleaners Film," *Screen*, Winter 1975–6, p. 101, for a particularly idealist account of straight cinema masquerading as oppositional).

Films in their construction can only make identification and the ideological power-positions of forms and contents of representation more, or less, problematic. Leaving a film feelii oneself a victim, as stated in the interview cited, is oppressior. not in each statistical case necessarily linked to physical rape. Additionally, in Western countries, one in seven females are victims of aggravated assault by men and/or rape before the age of seventeen, even according to the conservative *New York Times*. With such statistics accepted, one knows the incidence is far more extreme than that. The relations of voyeurism, rape, empirical statistics, bourgeois concepts of freedom of expression for maintaining male power, all coalesce here as questions problematized around the viewer-as-subject *through* the cinematic.

15   Lis Rhodes' *Light Reading* (1978)

Light Reading is an attempt at producing a different viewer and viewing through a different film. "This venture . . . both originates from, yet refuses containment by, existing discursive structures." (Nancy Woods, "On Light Reading," *Circles Distribution*, unpublished program notes, 1981–4).

"The film begins in darkness as a woman's voice is heard over a black screen. 'She' is spoken of as multiple subject – third person singular and plural. Her voice continues until images appear on the screen and then is silent. In the final section of the film she begins again, looking at the images as these are moved and re-placed, describing the piecing together of the film as she tries to piece together the tangle of strands of her story. The voice is questioning, searching. She will act. But how? Act against what? The bloodstained bed suggests a crime. . . . Could it be *his* blood – was that the action denied to Madame Beudet (in Germaine Dulac's 1922 *The Smiling Madame Beudet*)? No answers are given, after the torrents of words at the beginning all the film offers are closed images and more questions. . . . Is it even blood on the bed, what fracture is there between seeing and certainty? Could it be *her* blood –

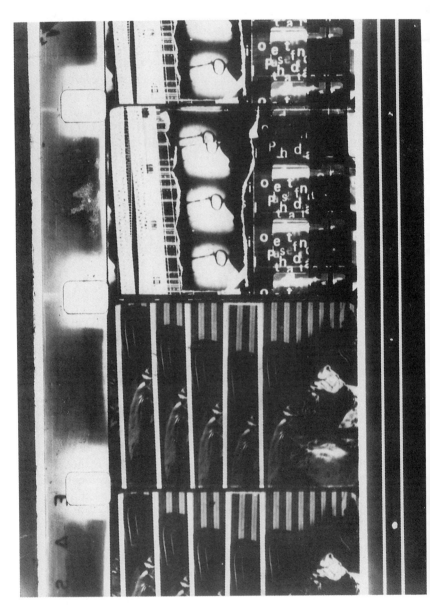

15 Lis Rhodes, *Light Reading* (1978)

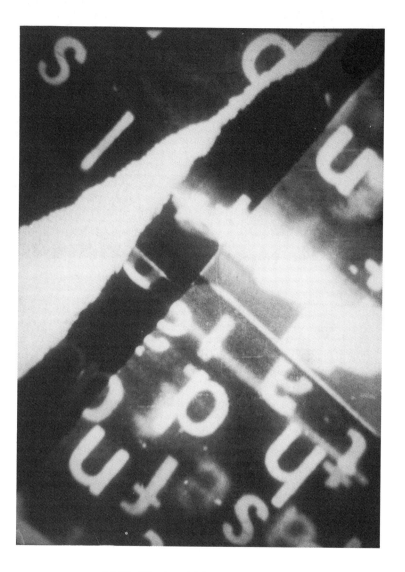

16 Lis Rhodes, *Light Reading* (1978)

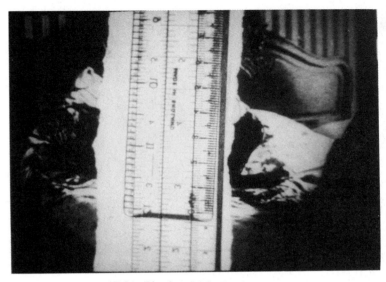

17 Lis Rhodes, *Light Reading* (1978)

rape, murder of the mind, of the body, of both? Her image has gone. If there has been a crime, 'she' might still be victim. . . . How can a crime of such complexity and continuity be 'solved'? The voice searches for clues, sifting through them, reading and re-reading until the words and letters, in themselves harmless enough, loom up . . . no longer hung on the structure of language. The clues suggest it is language that has trapped her, meanings that have excluded her and a past that has been constructed to control her. 'She watched herself being looked at, she looked at herself being watched, but she could not perceive herself as the subject of the sentence.' In *Light Reading* Lis Rhodes recognizes that dead-end. She searches for other clues and other means of finding her own reflection. But she seems to be framed everywhere she looks: the cosmetic mirror gives her back only part of her image, photographing herself in a mirror gives her back another. . . . She will not be looked at but listened to" (Felicity Sparrow, "*Light Reading*" in "Her image fades as her voice rises," Broadsheet, Arts Council of Great Britain, 1983).

"The film exceeds the present political boundaries of struc-

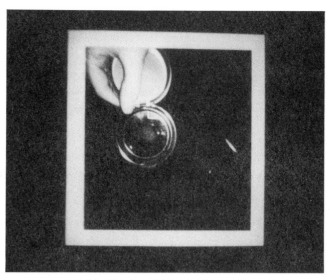

18 Lis Rhodes, *Light Reading* (1978)

tural/materialist filmmaking in harnessing this 'presentational strategy' [of the processes and materials of the film's construction] to a feminist critique of language and representation. The film invites a division into three sections. The first section consists of a black screen over which a woman's voice-over monologue is heard. The spoken text is related to the third person 'she'. We learn through the monologue that 'she' is alternately writing, reading, and attempting a story whose structure constantly eludes her: 'she saw the story in a moment . . . the end began where the beginning ended . . . inseparable in the myth of her memory and the sound of her voice . . . her hands reached out . . . she could only glimpse a shadow . . . the faint reflection of a fading image, slipping between the shadows, stumbling on the traces of her knowledge, sinking in the ruts of her experience . . . she couldn't reach herself . . . she begins again . . . and now she wrote . . . and now . . . the sense of the story is . . . is . . . but which moment of beginning follows which moment of end? . . . is the end beginning or the beginning ending? . . . She is told the end is not the beginning . . . if it were, she is told, how could she know the which from the witch, or the which from the why' (Lis Rhodes' text of *Light Reading* quoted from *Heresies*, no. 16, Film Issue, 1983, p. 88; Woods, op.cit.).

"The refusal to consider women as a class and to consider men as the antagonistic class relates back finally to its 'unthinkability.' If we dig a bit at these unthinkables we will notice that they themselves relate back to the set of confused representations which turn around the belief that there must necessarily be close and permanent relations between most females and most males at all times. This makes a structural conflict 'dysfunctional,' hence unthinkable. But it might be said that this is a question of reality, not of a 'belief.' But this 'reality,' or this 'belief' – the belief that such is reality – is not only ideological, but is the very heart of the ideology (i.e. of the representation of the world which supports the partriarchal system). There obviously also, there *above all*, the ideology does not appear as ideology but as the reasonable presentation of reality, as reality itself" (Christine Delphy, "A materialist feminism is possible," *Close to Home*: *A Materialist Analysis of Women's Oppression*, Hutchinson, London, 1984; University of Massachusetts Press, 1985, p. 180).

I will continue to use Nancy Woods' important essay to raise the film-theoretical questions *Light Reading* demands.

"In *Light Reading*, 'her' encounter with language, it would seem, is immediately confronted with the presence of an already existing structure proscribing the terms of her entry into discourse. This structure is easily recognized as that of narrative – the imperative of a beginning, middle, and end seemingly justified by the cause and effect relation it constructs. Any attempt to interrogate narrative logic and the rigidity of its structure is challenged with being itself illogical.

"[Yet] the monologue continues [on the sound-track]: '. . . the scene of her dream is disturbed by the present of a past not past . . . the past that holds her with fingers turned on logic . . . nails hardened with rationality . . . cutting the flow of her thought, forcing her back within herself . . . damned by the rattle of words . . . words already sentenced . . . imprisoned in meaning . . . exhausted with explanation . . . shot with pins of punctuation. . . .' The enforced marginality of women in meaning-production, and their subsequent confrontation with a hermetically sealed universe of discourse is traced to the imposition of a particular set of categories – those of Western rationality and logic – onto discourse. The status narrative enjoys as a privileged discursive mode is precisely because its investments in linear and instrumental relations conforms to the requisites of these categories. . . .

"The 3rd person 'she' drives a wedge between the voice and the text being read/heard/written, a wedge between the filmmaker and the material of film; this is a product of the work of both the unconscious fragmentary languaging and the conscious polemic, attempt to construct a position for the speaker, however anonymous that speaker may be, to the point where the speaker is reducible to nothing but the spoken" (Woods, op.cit.).

Gertrude Stein, H.D., and Samuel Beckett as valid precursors have used the "she" or "her" of such literary work – that aspect of the film, only momentarily isolated here, that can be called literary.

As to *Light Reading's* sound/image hierarchies, the aural attention of the spectator is primarily activated and engaged. "One consequence of this formal manoeuvre is the radical undermining of sight as the essential condition of the film's immediate intelligibility. This tactic precipitates a temporary shift of emphasis in the sensory registers by which film spectatorship is usually experienced, forcing the spectator to reconsider her/his habitual subjugation of sound to image." More correctly it is not a shift of registers from the usual experience of film, but rather producing in the spectator a *realization of the habitual subjugation of image to sound*. Here the film produces itself as such, whereas conventionally cinema represses this operation in the interests of narrative functioning, both in fiction-films and documentaries. Image is always subjected to sound, which is why you can put almost any soundtrack "over" any image and the resulting confluence will produce itself as "naturally" cohering with the sound. In this way, meaning is given by the sound's determinations.

The use of the compact mirror in *Light Reading* increasingly shifts its position until it returns a direct look to the camera/spectator. This is also what occurs in Warhol's *Kitchen*. There, characters in and outside of the film are constantly almost "caught," held in by the reflection of the mirror played with by Edie Sedgewick. We know that the mirror is capable of capturing/framing an image from outside the film-scene, however unacceptable an occurrence this might be. A tension is set up precisely because of the mirror's capacity as active term, rather than mere reflector of that which is given as correct and purposeful. Edie's playing with the mirror in *Kitchen* reflects from within the space, alluding to a without (camera crew or audience: differing times and spaces). The viewer's projection into that space becomes problematized as Edie's mirror-reflector wavers from the interior space to the camera-lens and viewer to those behind. Film thus as learning instrument, a didactic procedure presented, through anarchic play, a dialectic in film as to its possibilities to transform "the natural" scene, breaking the homogeneity. In *Light Reading* the image of the mirror functions similarly, as an ineluctable reflection of something *else*, disturbing any imagined closures including those of "the" something else. Functioning becomes disturbed. The natural consistently capitulates to labour.

"In *Light Reading*, stills are increasingly altered, now appearing defaced and marked. Finally the agent of this change is made explicit as a pair of hands enters the frame and (they) continue manipulating the various materials (photos, strips of film, rulers, scissors) which are consistent elements of the film's commitment to the structural/materialist imperative that the filmmaker literally make her/his role in the production process explicit. But it also anticipated a prominent concern for the final section, the inscription of the female body in representation" (Woods, op.cit.).

The structural/materialist imperative is slightly more complex, as it is not one demanding the documentation of the filmmaker's literal role in the production. Rather, it is the imperative of a process of pro-filmic (that which the camera is aimed at) and filmic transformations, through the viewer. A crucial distinction follows: the film as "record" of its own making and the modernist/post-modernist contingencies of such, must not be understood as some kind of *record-of*, but rather as the abstract of that. In the concrete empirical sense this does *not* mean a film that *documents* the filmmaking techniques via what we are given to see by the illusionist capacities of the photochemical recording device (film). Rather, it means film's abstract, a filmic real in which a process is instituted *as* a process, not the documentation *of* a process. A process of its own contradictions of presentation/representation, reproduction/effacement, attempted narrativizational hold of the spectator/impossible narrativizing of the spectator. The object *film* thus does not somehow essentially, or even momentarily in its operation, record an activity of something *else* and adequately represent that, but rather, complexly does not annihilate processes engaged. This is how "record of its own making" must be understood. A *radical* sense of Realism. Such a film is not about some other real, but is its Real.

The voice interrogates

"*Light Reading's* commitment to the structural/materialist imperative that the filmmaker literally make her/his role in the production process explicit . . . anticipates . . . the final section's inscription of the female body in representation." The concept of the document has been critiqued above; equally to be critiqued is the notion that the film inscribes the female body. "In the second and final monologue, this time in conjunction with an image track, we hear a highly self-reflexive recounting of the film's construction. Yet as well as offering a literal description of the place of editing cuts, footage lengths of sequences, camera movements, the voice interrogates how 'she' is implicated in the filmic structure which is emerging. What assumptions have been governing the film's organization?" (Woods, op.cit.).

". . . she was working back to front, front to back . . . images before thought . . . words proscribing images, images proscribing sounds? . . . which was in front of why? . . . was it just the orientation of her look, the position of her perception?" (Rhodes, "*Light Reading*," op.cit.).

So what is given is a series of questions, neither a sound-track answering or documenting the process, nor an inscription of the female body, fetishizing it and reintegrating the absent presence of the filmmaker. This film does not reintroduce such regressions for film or for the viewer. "She will not be looked at but listened to" (Rhodes, op.cit.). "This inquiry prompts closer reflection on a set of concerns specific to the feminist filmmaker, the film ending with the refusal of the particular status of 'objecthood' that patriarchal cinematic representation confers" (Woods, op.cit.).

". . . she looked more closely, she read more clearly . . . she saw that she was both the subject and object . . . she was seen and she saw . . . she was seen as object . . . she saw her subject . . . for what she saw as subject was modified by how she was seen as object . . . she objected . . . she refused to be framed . . . she raised her hand . . . stopped her action . . . she began to read . . . she began to re-read . . . aloud" (Rhodes, op.cit.).

Nancy Woods ends her essay as follows: "I have tried to argue that *Light Reading* exceeds the parameters of structural/materialist filmmaking in its articulation of feminist concerns. . . . Certainly even amongst avant garde film audiences, structural/materialist films continue to be categorized as difficult, inaccessible, boring, etc, thereby returning the responsibility for this marginal status to the films themselves. While the political/theoretical analysis which sustains structural/materialist views of spectatorship might be challenged, along with other tenets of the enterprise as a whole, this prematurely forecloses what is in question, namely the particular demands structural/materialist films make of their audience. Though avant garde enthusiasts readily elevate the Brechtian formulae of 'pleasure through instruction' to an almost prescriptive norm, the sometimes acute discomfort experienced in structural/materialist film, from which it seems at times that all familiar pleasure has been purposefully evacuated, is less warmly received. . . . *Light Reading's* own formal strategy – the extended use of black leader, the rejection of even the barest narrative thread, and the rigorous presentation of filmic materials and processes – may stand equally condemned on these grounds. However more is at stake in the project than a gratuitous assault on the collective psyches of spectators. As Stephen Heath has argued, 'The disunity, the disjunction, of structural/materialist film, is, exactly, the spectator. What is intended, what the practice addresses, is not a spectator as unified subject, timed by a narrative action, making the relations the film makes to be made, coming in the pleasure of the mastery of those relations, of the positioned view they offer, but a spectator, a spectating activity, at the limit of any fixed subjectivity, materially inconstant, dispersed, in process, beyond the accommodation of reality and pleasure principles.' "[12]

Light Reading is the possibility of a new direction for film, not to be co-opted by an overriding definition.

16 Questions around structural/materialist film

The argument continues in respect of the impossibility of history, or rather, its fundamental possibility only within narcissistic psychoanalytic structures, the historicizations thus of an ego-centered spectator in desire of control over object and spectacle. In such a definition the spectator is in endless transcendental self-identification and identification with the camera as fetishized metaphor for (patriarchal) self. Equally "impossible" for a radically materialist practice is an "other" history, as Stephen Heath argues: "If the history of cinema is radically impossible, two courses seem open: either the end of cinema as the straight refusal to make films and so repeat its terms or the end of cinema in films, a work in, on, through film, the 'truly materialist practice' as Gidal defines it. Such a practice . . . is then necessarily the fully reflexive knowledge of the history of cinema that at any moment a film – a materialist film – must hold and present, 'a dialectically constituted "presentation" of film representation, film image, film moment, film meaning in temporalness, etc.'. The film must be the event of that material presentation – ('the historical moment is the film moment each moment') the only way to end the implications of cinema, the place-image, identification, narrative-sign, illusion – of the spectator there" (Stephen Heath, "Afterword," *Screen*, Summer 1979).

"In one crucial sense at least, it is quite the reverse of the arbitrary that has to be stressed; historical materialism indeed is the science of the non-arbitrariness of the given, including meaning(s)" (ibid.). Heath's critique is incorrect. It is based on a base/superstructure homology, the real reflection of reality equalling *cinema*. Christine Delphy too stresses ideology as ideology-*of* – when it is not necessarily idealist to say ideas beget ideas. She is correct to state that ideology is not totally autonomous as a discourse, but physical reality, concrete material reality, is equally not totally autonomous. That is why the concept of semi-autonomy is so important. It is idealist to hope for more! She attacks the notion of "ideology its own cause," stating that "to accept this is to fall back into a theory of culture as totally arbitrary." But culture is totally arbitrary, as are the identities placed on the physical bodies of "male" and "female," as she argues so lucidly and consequently. Heath makes the same error of seeing historical materialism as necessarily "the science of the non-arbitrariness of the given." It is not. The given is determined but arbitrary. Socially, sexually, economically determined does *not* mean "non-arbitrary." Because all determinations are politically *constructed* (from nothing, i.e. not from any natural truth, essence, or even "in the last instance" from the physical. No more than a mind–body homology does the mind–body dualism get us anywhere, theoretically or politically). Certain determinations, like the end of capitalism not to mention the end of patriarchy, constantly have new agendas set. Although determined, their constructions transform in and through history. *Change.* Perhaps the "way out" of this contradiction is in the theoretical opposing of "the final" versus "the strategic." But "the final" itself is an ideological concept which disallows productive contradiction and struggle, and would thereby pre-empt, i.e. find an "answer" at the expense of, precisely, dialectical and historical materialism. The misunderstanding is thus of the concept *the arbitrary*. It simply does not mean that nothing has a relation to anything else, or that once meanings are produced they are "free" from material political/ideological interests. On the contrary, those determined constructions are arbitrary, as arbitrary as the decision of what a little boy or girl should "become." In that sense, the arbitrary and the ideological coincide, where one is "always already *for*. . . ."

With the endless attempts to privilege the phallus as primary signifier, by those defending Lacan (and most of psychoanalysis), and the endless attempts to privilege "sexual difference" (i.e. difference from), similarly, a concept of the arbitrary must be, with however much difficulty, and against however much resistance, instituted.

Thus, "historical materialism is the science of the non-arbitrariness of the given, including meaning(s)" only if one forgets dialectics, materialist politico-aesthetics. Take a photograph of a dead body. Take another of a knife. Those two images can function as pro-Nazi or anti-Nazi. The production of meaning, when it is solidified, in the way those images are put, can position one in one direction. That, though, does not then mean that those conjunctions are not arbitrary/ideological, but that they are.

Those meanings, images, words, still arbitrary, can function as the specific effect of a cause, or the specific effects of various causeless elements. That is their use for political struggles and meanings. *The production of meaninglessness in representational practice functions exactly to process such a position.* Thus film producing meaninglessness *does* (*pace* Heath) mean "in meaning, crossed by meanings, those of the history of cinema they inevitably and critically engage included – and productive of meanings, not least the complex meaning of their, of that, engagement" (Heath, op.cit.).

17 Meaning and illusion

Meaning and illusion function synonymously, in "a totally un-Brechtian manner," if Brecht is incorrectly understood as historicizing practice. The misunderstanding of Brecht, and his own contradictory formulations on the subject of representation's effects, ("thinking whilst crying . . . *political tears*") has been voluntarized to reduce Brecht-in-cinema to "films with modernistic style touching on important social issues." Such an all-purpose rationale leads to a broadened, rather than a reduced, concept of experimental cinema. The silly results of this are that, according to New York's *Village Voice*, "Tarkovsky, Syberberg, perhaps Chantal Akerman, and the Martin Scorsese of *Raging Bull* (are) avant garde features, on a budget of more than peanuts" (*Village Voice*, 3 May 1983). Such positions have become standard in *Screen*, *Frameworks*, *October*, and *Camera Obscura* as well as in all French and German film journals.

In order *not* to broaden but to reduce the concept of experimental film, meaning and illusion are to be problematized in the anti-illusionist project of a materialist cinema. Equally, just because the abstract is unrepresentable is no reason to use metaphor as a stand-in for it. It is useless to try for "historical specificity" via the metaphor, as if the latter were somehow more concrete an image, more real a symbol, than the abstract and general. Representing the abstract and general is impossible! But this ought not to legitimate metaphor under the guise of its being "specific." Of course, specifics of economics and politics and sexuality *can* be represented through the metaphor, but in that very way a decoy is established. A film "about" a rent-strike needs to annihilate the general principles which could be argued for 300 pages and deduce from one given, via metaphor, a total world of political meanings. This then denies both the materiality of the filmic process *and* the political specificity at hand *and* the abstract/general theories-positions taken on. Specific historical meaning is always given, filmically, at the expense of materialist processes which produce meaninglessness, that is, which undermine the power of the pregiven "reality" and "truth" of a representation. Positions taken are hopefully due to politics not "truth." One ideology not another, rather than "free from ideology." The contradictory motor for political questions of cinematic representation has no solution outside an ideology which accepts that all struggle is ideological, whatever else it is. A structural/materialist cinematic ideology refuses the fixing of reality by photomechanical means of representation.

18   The close-up

The following will be an example, that is, a model of the way in which a cinematic usage can differ (based on the

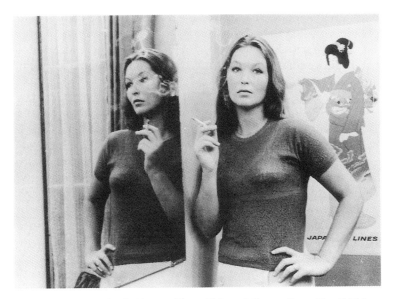

19 Jean-Luc Godard, *Two or Three Things I Know About Her* (1966)

transformations which it is formed by and which it forms) from "the rest" of the film it appears in. The way in which a close-up of, let us say, seventy-two frames' duration functions (three seconds at a normal speed of twenty-four frames per second) is grounded in the filmic context of each film. So meaning is formulated not only at the moment of the three-second sequence's being perceived by the viewer, or by its material existence as three-seconds of film-strip, but via its relation to the prior and forthcoming, and that in relation to the viewer's memory and rememoration attempts. Transformations are caused by memory and by the consciousness a reflexive process of attempted meaning-making demands. Thus the three-second strip here isolated for the purposes of this discussion must constantly be recalled within context.

The following, in addition to being a generalizable example, will be a definition of the way cinematic usage can differ in spite of its being the same device, here the close-up. The *use* is based on meanings which are culturally pre-constructed for us, in which we then construct.

From Godard's *Two or Three Things I Know About Her* (1966):
". . . long shot of the housing estate shopping centre, with
people hurrying to and fro. . . .
Commentary off screen: '. . . which according to the Minis-
try of Information communique, will give the Region a specific
and coherent orientation.'
Medium close-up of Juliette – Marina Vlady. Her back is
turned to the light and she appears to be standing on the balcony
of her own flat in the middle of the housing estate. Beyond, to
her left, another block of flats.
Commentary continued off screen: "That's Marina Vlady.
She's an actress. She's wearing a blue-grey sweater with two
yellow stripes. She's of Russian descent. Her hair may be light
or dark brown, I'm not quite sure which'.
MARINA parts her hair and stares into camera, then lowers
her eyes. MARINA: 'Yes, to speak as though one were quoting the
truth. Old Brecht said so. The actors must quote.'
Sound of children playing. New shot of Marina – Juliette
medium close-up, almost identical except that she now faces
the left-hand side of the screen while the block of flats in the
background is to the right.
Commentary continued off screen: 'She now looks right, not
that it matters. And it's Juliette Janson. She lives here. She's
wearing a blue-grey sweater with two yellow stripes. Her hair
may be light or dark brown, I'm not quite sure which. She's of
Russian descent.'
JULIETTE: 'Two years ago in Martinique. Exactly like in a
Simenon novel. No, I don't know which one. . . . Yes, *Banana
Tourists*, that's the one. I have to manage somehow. Robert
earns one hundred and thirty thousand francs a month, I think'
(old Francs – *ed*.). Commentary off screen: 'Now she turns her
head to the left . . . (*she does not turn*) . . . but it doesn't matter
. . . (*she turns her head to the left*)" (Jean-Luc Godard, *Screenplay:
"Two or Three Things I Know About Her*," (Lorrimer, London,
1975, pp. 123–4).
The close-up of Marina Vlady at the beginning of *Two or
Three Things* already is seen in relation to the title, thus the
ambiguity of the "Her." That there are, with Godard, often
two, or three, meanings, does not necessarily problematize any
of them. And problematization has to be established, cannot be

taken mechanistically for granted. When we see Vlady, and we think, due to our perceptions, that we "know" her (seeing is believing), this is not placed in contradiction, or doubt, simply because the "Her" of the title additionally happens to mean Paris. To make matters more unfortunate, the conflation of the city with the woman (*a* woman for Godard is always *woman*) itself is *not* the condensation of two separate meanings. It is thus not what Lacan would have called the condensation of signifiers (*Verdichtung*). It is already recovered, before any ambiguity could be set up. This conflation of woman and city is a deeply rooted patriarchal convention; conflation of the land, urban or rural, with woman.

So: ambiguity as such does not necessarily problematize meanings, as they are often separable and non-contradictory. And ambiguity itself is not instantiated by conflating woman, city, and the term "Her."

The third closure is that of "knowing." The viewer as voyeur, in the know, however partial and fragmentary, is still culturally given as knowing. An imperialist teleology becomes possible through the illusion of such partial knowing, each fragment building up a world from these bits. Building blocks of truth, colonized bit by bit, from perceptions, currents of knowledge, literary allusions, political desires, authors' fetishes, and so on. The dialectics of such fragmentary building can be reactionary or progressive, can be an idealist dialectics or a materialist one. Here is where the problem arises with this little example of three seconds of a close-up of a face in this Godard film. For how are these dialectics situated within the film and its diegesis, the narrative progression, the total mental, imaginary space of the film's continuum? And how is the viewer and the viewing dialecticized in relation to the representation? The commentary speaks: "She now looks to the right . . .", whilst she is looking to the left. The speaking refers to the stage-right, whilst she looks stage-left. Her position is thus given as the opposite of that which we assume to be meant, right and left from *her* position. Thus *what is given correctly is her movement from our position as viewers*. She is thus situated as the object of our discourse, natural to that. The viewer thus becomes identified with the filmmaker, or the omniscient *knower*. We are thereby given simply a larger frame, to include *us*. This is where the imperialization by the filmmaker–author comes in. We are also now geared up to expect parody and irony. The parodistic quality ("ah, she is facing in the opposite direction") for the viewer becomes an irony immediately ironed out as it is the dominant, accepted, code in which the actress performs. This works against an anti-illusionist practice in order to formulate the position of the woman as object and symptom. Vlady is acting for the unseen presence of the cinematic author, Godard, whose presence is invigorated precisely via her straight-into-the-camera eye-line match to that unseen presence: cameraman, director, viewer, and the identification-*through*. This is thus here no less necessitated than in the more conventional stylistics of the Hollywood narrative. The pro-filmic event is simply enlarged to include the unseen auteur, and his ramblings about the world, his amalgam of cultural–political references, literary bits and pieces, etc., as an illusionistically "more total" composite. The at one time Brechtian possibilities of quoting, reading, and speaking lines as if rehearsed, unnatural in their enunciation, here becomes a reification and fetishization. This becomes a suppression of the actress in the role enacted, stand-in for the author's unencumbered expression. Against this, the crux of a Brechtian theory of distanciation would have to be a dialectical subjectivity of the actress emplaced within, through, and against the author's text. In Godard's film, such Brechtian distanciation would be a threat to authorship.

The second oppression of the actress is the direct, imaginary, correspondence with the director. The close-up is made to verify the imaginary space of fiction film and the authority of patriarchal power for cinematic use. The viewer cannot but identify with this *as male*, thereby invisibilizing any non-male viewer and viewing. The position for women is against the viewer as male. The filmic system, any filmic system, is part of the cultural constituting of the viewer. It is through a Godardian practice that the spectre of change in cinematic reproduction is made untenable. (Not coincidentally(?) Godard the person remains proudly ignorant of the past decades' experimental films, surprising some. When asked about Michael Snow's work, Godard simply could not speak (*Camera Obscura*, 8/9/10, 1983, p. 176, transcription of a public debate in 1981).)[13]

"I never understood clearly what you Americans mean by

narrative or story. I was always accused of not having a story in my pictures and I always thought that if ever there was a picture with a story it was mine. A criticism I would make of critics is that they talk too much about the isolated characters and not about the movie itself" (ibid., p. 176). By "movie itself" Godard is referring *not* to the movie itself, but to the narrative, as is clear from the paragraph from which the sentence is taken.

To reiterate: whilst viewing Marina Vlady in *Two of Three Things*, the commentary speaks: "She's wearing a blue-grey sweater . . . her hair may be light . . . she turns her head to the left," etc. The viewer's position, via male identification, as holder of knowledge is reaffirmed, a position of (illusionary) superiority of viewer over viewed, and an ego-imposed coherence of understanding, including the understanding of parody, irony, contradictory information in image/sound, and so on. At the same time, the viewer's position in knowledge is as consumer manipulated into that illusion of mastery, *illusory* superiority, power over the objects that make up the object *cinema*. This calls for the obliteration via repression of the objective, and subjective, histories of the viewer, whilst under the rubric of mastery by said viewer. A seduction and oppression by conventional narrative and the stylistics of Godard, functioning as same. The conglomeration of facts and ideas and images from various discourses are subsumed to, and assumed by, a poly-historian. This is the position of the male in patriarchy. This placing of the viewer is what formulates the consistency of Godard's work, after *La Chinoise* (1967). The above example of the close-up in Godard is to be read against the following one, how the "same" usage can be, and can function as, different.

The close-up of Nico in *The Chelsea Girls* (Warhol, 1966) forms the first few minutes of that film. We see her framed in tight close-up. There is no eye-line match with an assumed viewer as in Godard's *Two or Three Things*. Rather, it is always a look slightly askew, perceived always as this nervousness in relation to the camera and audience. Through such deliberate avoidance of eye-line match (the actress's self-consciousness?) rather than Godard's form of clever "direct-address," the act becomes *act*. This difference matters, as any tension between "real feelings" and "acting" would evaporate given successful mimesis, once eye-line match to the assumed viewer is accomplished.

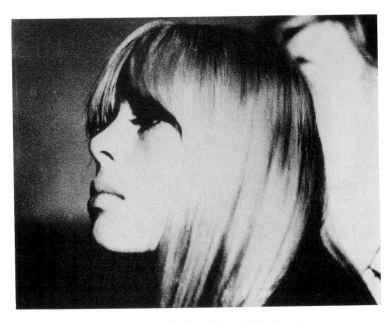

20 Andy Warhol, *The Chelsea Girls* (1966)

The opposite of such successful completion is apparent when Nico, in *Chelsea Girls*, remains in constant conflict through the nervously self-conscious avoidance of camera and crew presence within the space. A further dialectic tension is set up because all this can always be equally present as *acting*, as the enactment of this dialectic tension. But there is no insuring that this second reading could maintain itself in the face of the first, as somehow more true. The filmic thus is never settled once and for all, it has not become simply illustrative of a spatio-temporal irony.

Nico stares at the camera/viewer, slightly askew; she also looks away, into the (for the viewer) imaginary space recreated for the film, whether that be an actual kitchen or a kitchen set. This makes problematic the Nico face close-up sequence's instituting both documentary truth (looking, however askew, at the camera, thereby admitting its existence within the documentary apparatus) *and* simultaneously instituting fiction (her looking off into the room, speaking to someone off-screen, later on-screen . . . someone else?). And so on. This immediate

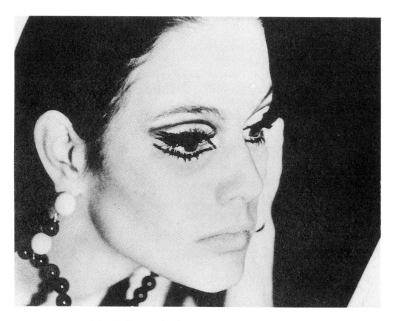

21 Andy Warhol, *The Chelsea Girls* (1966)

problematization of the viewer-position comes about because
of the said ambiguity, and because of the way the ambiguity
does *not* function to make of fiction versus documentary two
possible readings *both possibly right*. It also does not allow
mutually exclusive readings, one permitted its force as truth
simply dependent on which interpretation/reading is "chosen."
Rather, both are against the grain, constantly not given enough
validity to function as truth or as multiple possibilities somehow
sustainable and frozen. The ambiguity forces neither fiction
nor documentary to bring an imaginary adequacy; consumption becomes impossible, and the solidifying of the viewer's
collaboration becomes equally impossible. This is what begins
to constitute a negative practice: what is impossible, does
not sustain the viewer's culturally induced desires, does not
reproduce certain illusions of power over meaning, does not
allow meaning to view itself as ahistorical, etc. Equally, this is a
practice which produces a viewer of necessity questioning and
questioned. What is my place in this? Am I in this at all? Am
"I" in this at all? The viewer is part of the cinematic apparatus.

The close-up in *Chelsea Girls* forces such a function. This three minutes' sequence demands a different and differing viewer, one not posited idealistically, and mechanistically, separate from his or her history, memory, wants, thoughts, etc. The unconscious too has its, your, history, which here is not suppressed by narrative's "needs".

The reproduction of the viewer is always in relation to those histories. In that sense, materialist practice is defined through redundancy, i.e. the viewer is in history by being a viewer, as opposed to being a voyeur, the latter being a state which necessitates the repression of any reflexion (though unconscious fear of being caught substantiates the tension). The viewer is in history, and the attempted representation/reproduction of the pro-filmic in cinema is in history because the photochemical trace can never be outside history, because *nothing is outside of history*. The same goes for the viewer. Yet other cinemas function outside history by giving themselves *as if* they were outside history. And when the viewer is set up as voyeur, it is the positing of a view *as if* he/she could be outside history.

Another way of stating this is that Warhol's use of the close-up in *The Chelsea Girls* sequence described tells the viewer that he/she does not know. To know what or that you don't know. The close-up functions similarly in *13 Most Beautiful Women* (1964), in spite of the latter's being empirically more similar to the Godard. In *13 MBW* each "portrait" lasts for three and a quarter minutes, at silent speed. Each is a head staring back and determinately not doing so. A line is given, from your eye through the camera-person('s), through the camera-lens, to the subject to be identified, identified into, having become the subject/object of your viewing. The subject/object looking back, you now become the subject/object of hers. Yet the line of viewing is problematized. Objects of her gaze (unseen by the viewer) are within and without the framed enclosure. Act and action are minimalized; such film is a prefiguration of structural/materialist film which relinquishes any look back. In *13 MBW* the question is still am I, viewer, behind and through the camera-eye (and filmmaker) identified (via the apparatus, or by myself in narcissistic self-identity) imaginarily in seen or unseen space? In *13 MBW* the voyeuristic camera stare still premises a stare back.

Instructions for split-screen Projection of Andy Warhol's THE CHELSEA GIRLS

Projector No. 2 Left	Projector No. 1 Right
	Right projector begins the film with Reel no. 1 'NICO IN KITCHEN'
	Play for five minutes alone with sound, then turn sound down until just audible below reel no. 2
Reel no. 2 'POPE ONDINE AND INGRID'	
Begin only after five minutes of reel no. 1 and continue with sound until beginning of reel no. 3	
	Reel no. 3 'BRIDGIT HOLDS COURT'
Reel no. 4. 'BOYS IN BED'	Begin with sound as soon as threaded. Cut sound on reel no. 2
No sound	
	Reel no. 5 'HANOI HANNAH'
Reel no. 6. 'MORE HANOI HANNAH & GUESTS'	All sound
No sound until reel no. 5 goes off	
Leave sound on while threading reel no. 7 and then turn off sound and begin sound on reel no. 7	
	Reel no. 7 'MARIO SINGS TWO SONGS'
Reel no. 8 'MARIE MENCKEN'	Sound until female impersonator exits which is approx-imately the first ten minutes. Then off
Colour	
Sound only after reel no. 7's sound is off	
Play until end of reel	
	Reel No. 9 'ERIC SAYS ALL'
Reel no. 10 'COLOR LIGHTS ON CAST'	Colour
Colour	All sound after end of sound on reel no. 8
No sound	
	Reel no. 11 'POPE ONDINE'
Reel no. 12 'NICO CRYING'	All sound
Sound for the last ten minutes under reel no. 11	
After no. 11 end, turn light off on no. 12 but continue sound as exit and intermission music	

General notes:
As soon as a reel ends, it sould be replaced immediately by the next one scheduled for that projector and then begun at once. However, a five-minute difference is intended between the two projectors, to be established at reel no. 2, and the projectionist should pause, if necessary, to maintain this interval.

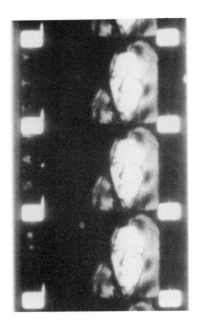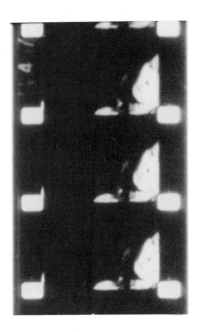

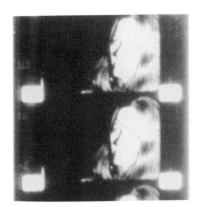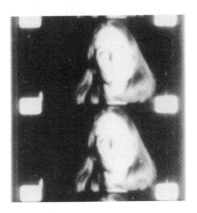

22 Andy Warhol, *13 Most Beautiful Women* (1964)

19 Context

Contexts change. No work is separable from context; its meanings always function within it, which is precisely why it is an idealism to try to isolate specifically made up viewer-contexts, isolating viewers for example who think x rather than y, allowing their individualistic "collectivity" to determine a text's meanings. That would be to assume that a material text had no social force, was simply always again an effect of a particular interpretation brought about *a priori* by this or that happenstance group of "subjects" who each time make a "new" context which thereby permits new ideas. Such an idealist position sees groupings of individuals, misnamed "context," producing the world from their individualities. The best example I know of this perversion is the notion argued that film x is a parody of film y. When it is pointed out that film x was made seven years before film y, and therefore could not be a parody of it, the reply is, "But I, and the other viewers, didn't know that, therefore it *is* a parody." This is how rampant individualism is entitled context.

20   History

"Has any materialist account ever proceeded by tautology?" (Stephen Heath, "Afterword," *Screen*, Summer 1979, p. 99). This question must respect the formulation enunciated two pages before: "an obsessive engagement with staring and staring back, predicated on a materialism of the specific historical moment, each moment."

The solipsism, everything is historical therefore this is, must be answered. But it cannot be answered by reintegrating "significance," historical significance or other, with a represented/representable content; significance otherwise becomes attached to a concept of adequately representable *specific historical truth*. "Because the cinematic apparatus certain films use is not just material, or pure machinery, but an integral part of an institution of representation, transformation of the elements of that institution cannot remain merely formal, but must produce and imply transformation of the content of the representations, and of their attitudes to the institution, and of our attitudes as spectators at the same time" (Ben Brewster, "Notes on Film," *Perspectives on British Avant Garde Film*, Arts Council of Great Britain, Hayward Gallery, London, April, 1977, unpaginated). This realizes that a naive need to have a preconstituted subject-matter that is correct for avant-garde/experimental film practice on the Left would deny the historicity of objective film-processes. Such objective film-processes must ignore the individual choices of "opportune" pro-filmic events, otherwise significance becomes reintegrated, attached to some preconceived historical truth.

An example of such a reintegration is the way the specificity of history is by some seen to reside in the car-sequence "Driving through Rome" in Straub/Huillet's *History Lessons* (1974). Whatever the Brechtian motives for a dialogue in new Rome about old Rome, its interspersion with the drive through the city streets simply gives "significance" to the enacted street-sequences, alternating with those of actors wearing robes from 194 BC, sounds of honking car horns overlaying the latter. This distanciates in a most academic fashion, questioning neither the veracity of the present-day Rome nor the faithful fiction 194 BC. And the film is basically formed from these two sequences. This is a Godardesque mechanization of significance via the *seen*. Here perception equals knowledge, instead of being questioned by it. Attached to this conceptual misfortune is "the historical." Such a representation of history, past or present, or past and present, is (the filmmakers'?) *imaginary* given as truth (dialectical or not).

This is how deconstruction is instanced. A minor matter is that this deconstruction is additive, Metzian/Derridean/Burchian deconstruction subtractive. In other words, instead of one shot negating, or distancing, the previous one, thereby (so the argument goes) questioning the narrative codes utilized, here in the example from *History Lessons* we have the additive deconstruction, one scene lumped upon the previous in Godardian, but naively simplified, fashion. Ostensibly this is to distance the straightforward documentariness and fictiveness of each representation, yet what occurs is that document and fiction become ideologically instanciated as equal powers moving the truth of an illusion in the direction of representation's adequacy, "reality" or "political truth." In a sense this "positive deconstruction" is Metzian/Derridean/Burchian deconstruction minus (even) the latter's pessimism. Thus the former becomes a sentimental humanism of progress.

So the question is one of how to historicize without formulating a phantasm of documentary truth or concomitant deconstruction. The *only* possible manner of approach is to utilize the question of cinematic representation as a historical question. So the solipsism again: it is historical because it is. The radical problematization of, and taking issue with, historical film forms *can* be through the filmic, against the various metadiscourses being operated.

A discourse can be materially historical, without needing a metadiscourse to place it into "historical perspective." What is equally needed is theory, whether lagging behind practice or not. This analogy with the way filmic practice does not have to build in a perspective of historicization is important, so as not to formulate a theory, knowingly or not, predicated upon the needs of metadiscourses to frame, give perspective to, and finally justify practices.

"There is for Gidal a radical impossibility: the history of cinema. The fundamental criticism made of everyone from the Berwick Street 'Collective' to Ackerman, Oshima, to LeGrice (even LeGrice) is that their films are part of that history, return its representation, that they are in that cinema, repeat its implications. Strategies of deconstruction are merely a further turn of involvement: deconstruction repeats – gives currency once more to and looks into – the terms, the images it seeks to displace, is a continuing and reactionary reproduction of cinema. And cinema is not available here for another – alternative – history. It is inconceivable that Gidal could write a book such as LeGrice's *Abstract Film and Beyond*, the different, hidden, outside-the-industry, independent history. There is always in Gidal's writing the tension of an acute actuality, the pressure of – *for* – a break now, exactly the constant current *impossibility*" (Heath, "Afterword" op.cit., p. 94).

What such a critique of history forgets (and this relates to a forthcoming example of the way in which a splice operates via a loop structure, or not) is that the current impossibility produces by fits and starts history from the impossible, but also does not. To communicate is impossible, and those writers who refuse to know this and theorize it and process it are writing nineteenth-century novels (bad ones) dressed up as (at best) something slightly different. This does not mean that, in the face of communication's impossibility, speech is impossible. There is and is not independence from dominant history: thus no completely separable "independent history" but a history nevertheless of experimental practices, influences, relations. *And* "there is no history" if by *history* is meant a work always already implying the concrete material meanings and positions of its future. Rather not be in history if that means always already taking a role which history has conveniently left open to be specifically taken, in a certain required manner, in certain interests. Against that, certain experimental/avant-garde film *produces* history. That is why some films must be dealt with as they exist *as projected*, problematically, radically, with great difficulty in their opposition and "impossibility."

21   The literal

In the *Chelsea Girls/Two or Three Things I Know About Her* examples, "bad sound" in the former makes synchronization function as out-of-synch. In the latter, speech is always found in synch, synchronicity is never lost, even when a sound/image construction signifies and refers to itself, i.e. the apparatus cinema, or the ostensible filmmaker in the imaginary space, present in absence. The so-called "natural" homogeneity of sound with image is a base which remains the convention, in the Godard. Thus, any disturbances created for the viewer in the latter are literary, against *Chelsea Girls'* literal*ness.

Chelsea Girls could be called a "poor cinema;" a literalist roughness of process is here what transforms meanings. Out-of-synch in Godard (if such existed) would be conceivable as slick disjunction, both sound and image still retaining its

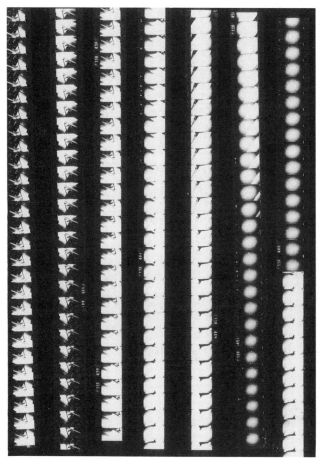

23 Peter Gidal, *Room Film 1973* (1973)

meanings, its (exchange) values within the scene of spectacle, never grating, clawing, difficult. Difficult dialectics opposed to smooth dialectics. There's so much immediate pleasure in the one it must be suspect.

A further example of the literal: Deke Dusinberre has written as to *Room Film 1973* (*Structural Film Anthology*, British Film Institute, 1976): "The play of surface and of substance becomes crucial to the film. For it is not merely a film about light and the absence of light (the white-out ending arrives after several

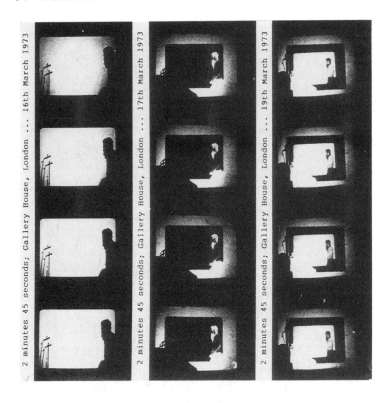

24 William Raban, *2 Minutes 45 Seconds* (1973)

extended periods of blackness) but about how insubstantial light can evoke substantiality. Roughly halfway through the film the image of a potted plant is seen, in a close-up concentrating on the leaves. The image is recognizable and, as such, bears some (illusory) substance. But as extreme close-up alternates with one less close, the viewer loses the ability to discriminate between the plant and the shadow it casts on the wall behind it; the shadow has as much visual substance as the image of the object itself. This ploy is amplified when, toward the end of the film, the plant is seen again in close-up, with its shadow again playing an important visual role. This time, the camera zooms out into a rare medium shot to reveal a mirror. The object and the shadow of that object and the reflection of both are situated on the same level of image-insubstantiality within the film. Thus *Room*

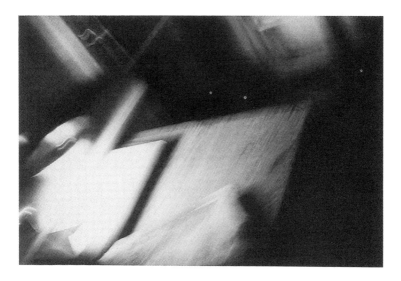

25 Peter Gidal, *Close Up* (1983)

Film 1973 attempts to exploit the representational proclivities of cinematography while continually denying representation by exposing the illusion on which that representation rests.

"As described above, then, the film deals with the issue of cinematic representation on a rather literal level; despite its concern with light as a primary element in that representation, *Room Film 1973* is not comfortably receptive to an analysis which presents it as a neo-platonic consideration of the nature of light. That critical tactic, in fact, would be typical of the American critical practice which has accompanied the North American structural films. Those films are open to analyses which involve an analogic principle, a principle which assumes that the structure of the film serves not only to elaborate the cinematic system of representation, but also serves as an analogue for other systems of meaning. Thus crucial structural films are seen as, say, an analogue for the rejuvenation of vision (*Tom Tom the Piper's Son*), or as an analogue for a Gnostic epistemology (*Zorns Lemma*) or as a metaphor for the intentionality of consciousness (*Wavelength*). It would seem, too, that the larger tradition of American avant-garde filmmaking has exploited such analogic

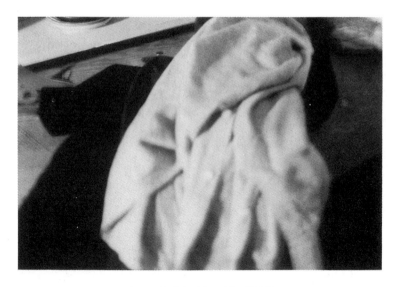

26 Peter Gidal, *Close Up* (1983)

techniques – primarily that of the metaphor, in which the formal concerns of filmmaking are conflated with another perceptual or epistemological or philosophical problem. But what has made structural films eminently receptive to this tradition is that *their dominant shape or structure automatically suggests modes of organization and meaning other than purely filmic ones* [italics mine].

"This analogic strategy has enabled North American structural films to neatly supersede the dilemma posed by *Room Film 1973*. That dilemma concerns the formalist aspect of modernism ('formalism' is being used here in a casual, non-pejorative context to refer to films which privilege the formal concerns of the medium over any content; historically, the filmic avant–garde has been generally formalist, but it has become a specific concern since the ascendance of the structural film). Formalism strives to render visible those formal postulates which are used "transparently" by the dominant practice of the medium. Obviously, the formal devices of dominant cinema are not always completely transparent/invisible – hence 'stylization' – but a stylized form is ultimately subordinated to the demands of the dominant practice. The formalist project is to challenge

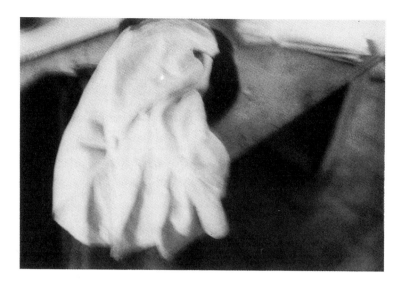

27 Peter Gidal, *Close Up* (1983)

the coherent system of formal practices which subtend the dominant practice and thereby challenge the organization of meaning and, ultimately, the entire system of signification established by the dominant practice. It does this by separating the formal postulates from their conventional context and revealing the way in which they operate, the way in which they determine representation. The putative rationale for this activity is not merely to regenerate a variety of representational forms, but to challenge the very ideology which founds its representation of reality on that system of signification.

"The dilemma which eventually arises with a rigorous formalist practice is that by making the processes of representation progressively arbitrary (so that those processes become, as it were, underdetermined rather than overdetermined) it runs the risk of lapsing into meaninglessness. For any system of meaning-making demands a differentiation – if not hierarchicization – of signifiers, so that when formalism assaults that system without suggesting an alternative system, it approaches a state of entropy and becomes – in terms of communication theory – 'meaningless'. . . . [But] to yield any insight into those processes of perception which determine cinematic presentation and representation, the formalist film must suggest another order of signification in addition to the one 'film is.' The dilemma, therefore, is that the formalist film must remain fundamentally reflexive, constantly challenging not only the dominant representational practice but also its own practice as that very representation is presented, *and* it must represent itself in a way which is continually 'meaningful.'

"North American structural films thus engage in the formalist project and simultaneously assure another level of meaning through the analogic approach. But recent English structural filmmaking is involved in an asceticizing strategy which makes the formalist dilemma more urgent. That is, it denies the analogic tactic and attempts to literalize the levels of meaning available to analysis of the film. The 'ascetic structural' films tend to minimize both content and analogic comparison by effacing – without completely abandoning – the representational image. They are also fundamentally 'shapeless'; the end of the film cannot be predicted, there is no 'goal' achieved, and there is *no overall shape which could be metaphorically exploited to engage other issues* [italics mine]. (Dusinberre, "The ascetic task," op.cit., pp. 110–12).

"What is interesting about *Room Film 1973* is the way it has literalized viewing experience without demanding a 1:1 correspondence . . . due to the erratic camera-movement which masks the precise repetition while suggesting a great repetitiveness as a whole. Despite the other tactics in the film which contribute to its visual impact – graininess, tinting, under-illumination, loss of edge of frame, etc. – it is the camera-work which remains most central in determining that impact. The camera not only contributes to the incoherence of the imagery, but also to the incoherence of the space. It never constructs a discrete space; that it was shot in one room remains an assumption on the part of the viewer. . . . It undermines the establishment of a unity of space just as it undermines (in editing) the unity of time, yet it struggles to maintain literalness of the recording and viewing experience.

"The erratic and often unfocussed use of the camera effectively yields a camera uninterested (or at least disinterested) in the objects it scans. The camera-movement is not mechanical, as is the editing procedure, but appears almost random or arbitrary. So that the film privileges the very process of configuration of the image on the part of the recording apparatus *and* on the part of the viewer; by making the perception of an image on the screen difficult and by rendering those images banal and almost 'meaningless,' the film rigorously reduces the semantic element and forces the spectator back onto her/his own capacities for meaning-making" (Dusinberre, op.cit., p. 113).

Thus Dusinberre argues for a practice which disallows to cinematic forms the analogic principle. This is so that, for example, a film process does not of necessity (and endlessly) have to become a metaphor for something else, analogue for another system of meaning, a universe of ideas or things referred to but unseen. Thus Dusinberre's emphasis on the literal. And yet, at the same time, he warns of a reductive film-as-film tautology. The only way through this is to problematize at each moment the relation between film procedure/film apparatus, and that which the camera is aimed at and attempts to reproduce. This point is argued further under the rubric that follows.

22   Artistic subject/aesthetic subject

"Since [this] formalist dilemma . . . in which radical formal strategies render the processes of representation so arbitrary that they run the risk of lapsing into meaningless tautology . . . ultimately implies a shift in the location of the responsibility for meaning-making, and since it has engaged – at one point or another – all of the modernist arts, it might be useful here to extend the notion of the subject to describe both the 'artistic subject' (the 'maker' – writer, filmmaker, painter, etc.) and the 'aesthetic subject' (the 'perceiver'); this makes clearer the idea of a general shift of meaning-making responsibility along an axis of subjects intersected by the art object . . . to reinscribe a *new* artistic voice [into . . . film] while escaping the cinematic solipsism exemplified by the films of Brakhage (just as Beckett had to

escape the solipsism implicit in an intensified authorial voice).
. . . A new and fragmented artistic subject . . . simultaneously
intensifying and contradicting a unified subjectivity to the point
of disintegration could only become clear though an analysis
recognizing neither the 'voice' of the theoretician nor the 'eye'
of the filmmaker as privileged or transcendent subject, but
insists on their inscription – on all levels – as operative factors
in theoretical and cinematic discourse" (Deke Dusinberre,
"Consistent oxymoron: Peter Gidal's rhetorical strategy," *Screen*,
Summer 1977).

23   Duration

Duration in printing/projecting in materialist film technically
shows aspects of (non)discontinuity. Rather than "continuity"
being posited as the given, it is really a matter of non-
discontinuity because duration, the piece of time presenting
itself filmically as duration (and inculcating in the viewer a
position of expectancy, for example, towards that duration,
cut at beginning and end by the splice) is not to be linked to
a continuum. The theoretical point taken here is that duration
and continuum have no necessary links, any more than the
previously discussed one to one relation of film to viewer has
any necessary linkages. Thus, duration can be theorized in
relation to discontinuity, the piece of filmstrip-time which is
cut at begin and end by the splice. This occurs if the filming is
in such a way as NOT to deny duration. This *may* also persist as
duration when non-discontinuous, i.e. perception of continuous image. It is within such complex relations that a cinematic
piece of photochemical reproduction exists. Through that, *then*,
certain representings of "contents," certain preceding and
simultaneous and following editing devices, certain matters of
grain, light, movement, focus, determine the functioning as
materialist or anti-materialist, illusionist or anti-illusionist, and
so on. As Rose Lowder, a French filmmaker/theoretician
states it: "in the case of . . . we have a film that is politically
progressive but formally backward. I am willing to concede

that the authors had progressive intentions but do not think that a film can be to any purpose progressive and backward at the same time. Formally backward is still backward" (Rose Lowder, "Recent film problems," Avignon, February 1983, unpublished).

The aims of narrative and narrativization may suppress, or repress, or detour material durational functioning. Duration is qualified/quantified in each specific case, by the image and the camera movement. Quantity "becoming" quality, a Hegelian notion, is problematic in that a quantum of wantum (Beckett) certainly has its effects, but "quality" apart from being a spurious concept, does not actually emanate from quantity except in certain cases, murder becoming genocide, private property becoming ownership of the means of production, and so on.

Duration in printing, duration in projecting, technically shows aspects of non-discontinuity, producing the machine as the whole apparatus rather than its opposite: the specific fetish. Such a film-process, one piece of film, one length, with duration produced in relation to discontinuity rather than as a naturally posited continuum, allows for cinema to operate ideologically as an apparatus wherein all elements take part, and are part of, the process. This then is, in theoretical terms, posed *in contradiction to* the cinematic apparatus's "aspects," for instance aspects of the filmmaking and filmviewing process given as specific fetish, metaphor for something which is not, metaphor for a lack, or narrative *of* a lack.

Certain usages hold certain processes of film to the concept and reality of the fetish (bad enough!), and then to the current specifically overdetermined patriarchalized fetish-*meanings* (worse!). Underlying this slightly arcane and compulsive definition, it must be recalled that the metaphorical usage of the fetish, as described, maintains both to the filmic "content" (Gilda in *Gilda*) and to the filmic form (*inseparable from content*, i.e. form is content, nevertheless definitionally separate from content when content is the imaginary referred to – real or otherwise).

Fetish can also be conceptual, as in the notion of "efficiency," of a film having to give the illusion of completing some act, as if that were the only way to struggle against "art for art's sake." "The inability to deal with designifying works or semioticity-denying works arrives at a pseudo-apparatus close to Stalin's efficiency" (*The Cinematic Apparatus*, Macmillan, London, 1986, p. 132). Thus the matter of *duration* is not isolate. It is a theoretical concept, concrete, which operates in relation to film-meaning (filmmaking and filmviewing) determining thereby the politics of work for, or against, fetish meaning.

"600 shots, sea gulls, of varying lengths, speeds, scale, and tonality" (Lucy Panteli, "Notes for a film, *Across the Field of Vision*," London, January 1984, unpublished). "A similar referent from shot to shot (seagull against sky) constantly changing through filmic operations 600 shots varying length speed scale tonality from edit to edit each image serves to link one gesture to another never culminating at a given place or space within the frame or from shot to shot no connection

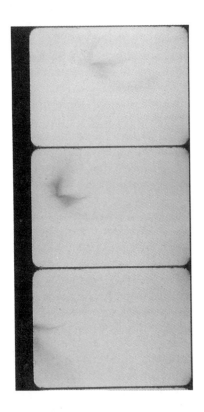

28 Lucy Panteli, *Beyond the Field of Vision* (1983)

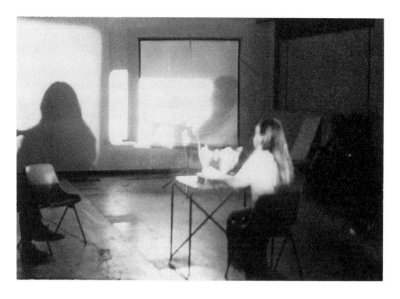

29 Annabel Nicholson, *Reel Time* (1973)

of sky to land no scale of distance outside of filmscreen not a
documentary around the theme of bird migration a registration
of comings and goings nonetheless into out of across a field of
vision an interplay of movement and positioning conditions of
expectations and reactions" (ibid.).

24   Splice

A splice mark is a photographic image, a reproduction, as
is every cinematic device, given through projection of film
through a projector. This is not an ontological inference but
rather a description of a determinate effect of a photochemical
process. Similarly, effects of cinema-technological operations
have certain meanings, though the technology, effects, meanings (or anything else) are not ontological. If they were they
would have to be avoided (voided) the way biologism has to
be, no matter what the state of any proof happens to be at

any time. This also dispenses with ethics, finally, so that good nature or bad nature ceases to matter. It ceases to be material. It is, precisely, material. Splice, producing itself as splice, makes of a shot of celluloid (acetate?) a material piece of time. To be situated as a viewer in relation to and engaging with, and processed by, and through, such a material piece of time means that the shot is materially enacted as *finite*. In the narratives of dominant cinema, a shot is always given as *infinite*. Thus it produces itself and the viewer through it as infinite, a realist/naturalist infinity, whether through metaphor or not. *This pertains to both space and time.* That is, the space given within the cohering rectangular frame, within that convention of seeing reality, is simultaneously given as if the convention were invisible, were in fact "transparent," so that the specificity of the rectangular convention, and the various codes necessarily operated to produce a viable narrative scene, or documentary representational sequence, is obliterated. In such a case, truth exists as if unencumbered by its having been produced via a production process. As if it could be communicated from its place to you directly. This invisibility of the conventions of cinema, the rectangle, perspective(s), eye-lines matching, and so on, including codes of sharpness, of peripheral (non)vision, and so on, allows the coherence of the scene. At the same time, its infinitude/eternitude is thereby *organized*. What this means is that, at the time of a particular scene, no other time, and no other space, from within the film (prior or forthcoming) or from without (from the realisms and the ideological realisms of the non-cinematic world) can engage the viewer. This operation of cinematic repression of time and space can be obliterated by the foregrounded splice, disallowing easy functioning of the cinematic machine, its illusions.

If one is nuts for psychoanalysis one could say the repression of the splice is the repression of castration, and thereby the repression of sexual difference, but this would not necessarily get one anywhere, as the necessity for acceptance of psychoanalytic models, themselves often "theorizations" based on this or that happenstance event, is problematic, more so when prescription is sold as description, and specific cultural oppressions are universalized thereby. Men utilize traditional metaphorical literary devices to reproduce their power, as in:

"Paternal signifier . . . without which . . . relations between the sexes impossible. It needs the voice of the master. The primary signifier, the phallus, is essential, without which no sexuality is possible." (Jacques Lacan, *Four Fundamental Concepts of Psychoanalysis*, Hogarth Press, London, 1977, p. 109). (Other) psychoanalytic models are not always wrong. And the theorization may prove productive without being "true." It is simply that the concept of the "true" must first be thrown out, as must be "the saintliness of the analyst" (Kristeva, quoted in "On Julia Kristeva," *Undercut*, no. 11, 1982). Then the questions of the usefulness *or otherwise* of making a link between the acceptance of "castration" (differently for the male, differently for the female) and the way a child is placed within an oppressive sexual (objective) history subjectively, *and film*, can be asked. If a splice is simply seen as "castrating" the true continuum of natural image, then it functions in as retrograde a manner as does in another, more supposedly conventional film, a "non-splice" (i.e. the hiding of the splice through codes of movement, story, and so on). Such a "non-splice" avows castration via vehement denial's unconsciously moti-vated component (and concomitant questionableness). Such a "non-splice" also avows castration and conventional sexual categories by placing the characters and the viewer in precisely the dominant sexual regime of meaning. A regime which allocates power and authority to the biological male.

What matters is the manner in which uses function, in each specific film at hand. No cinematic function can be ontologized, such as splice versus non-splice, or sound-over-image versus lack of it. Lenin warned that often mechanistic materialism is the greater danger, idealism the lesser, because the latter can still be dialectical and one has to educate away the idealisms, whilst the former is a mechanistic and undialectical basis for whatever formulations are made, theories constructed, politics avowed. Such mechanization is then harder to dialecticize, as it becomes the base for an entire method and practice, whatever the method (Lenin, *Materialism and Empirio-Criticism*).

In LeGrice's *Blind White Duration* (1968) the splice foregrounds the *de-repression of duration*. "This film takes to extreme a number of the specific ideas which emerged in the two films *Castle*

I, Castle II, and in *Talla*. Firstly, it is a film concerned with constructing an experience out of limited perceptions. The viewer is introduced to a limited range of images in short soft fade-ins and outs or quick flashes. Secondly, it is concerned with the light of the projector – the white screen and the white image which emerges out of it. The material was shot in the snow in January 1968. Thirdly it is concerned with repeats and near repeats in different sequential and superimpositional juxtapositions. Fourthly with the role of the viewer as a positive constructor of experience from the images. And fifthly with the use of unexceptional images which are not contrived in a studio or dramatic sense. I think this film might be seen as a more poetic and less dogmatic Vertov-like piece. Vertov himself predicted a kind of film which might have visual rhythms and poetic metre. Maybe this is a useful way of thinking about this film" (Malcolm LeGrice, London Film Co-op Catalogue, 1969 and 1974).

The meaning of the splice foregrounding the de-repression of duration is that various filmic devices repress the duration of a scene or sequence or piece of film-time. It is not simply a choice to do one thing or another, because each device is always already a cultural/social device within film history, and many a device has already been utilized within a number of films which operate differently from the specificity at hand. The viewer's positioning is never separable from that history, which is her or his social history of cinema and cinema-memory. At the same time, there is the apparatus of film which can be used for the *new*, for that which is specifically different. Alternative, counter, and oppositional independent cinema, if it is experimental, and if it is an avant-garde, is always already *against* that history. It is the splice, in *Blind White Duration*, which makes one question the difference between one image and another, and each's meaning. Such a questioning *inhibits* the free flow of desire/satisfaction. This means that such a work is continuously problematizing, and reflexive. Whilst the conscious is not thereby somehow eradicated, the concept *conscious* does not terminate in bourgeois rationalism. It is precisely problematic, not reductive or inductive. Without the work of the splice, in *Blind White Duration* the continuum established would be somewhat like a rather impressionistic

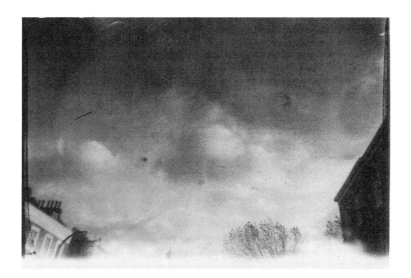

30 Roger Hammond, *Astigmatic* (1985–7)

subjectivist documentary of a space, kept unclear but searched *through*. (Un)fortunately no still could even hint at any of this. The profilmic, in other words, would automatically take precedence if the splices were either "absent" or produced in the way they usually are in narrative film, i.e. as invisible. In the series of loops making up the film *Berlin Horse* (LeGrice, 1971) the expectancy manipulation of fear and anxiety, which is constantly re-established through the loop of the burning horse/running horse image, becomes "the same" again and again. Yet it is never the same. The question of sameness thus only instantiates itself via the splice's intervention on the continuum of documented action or, in the case of *Blind White Duration*, inaction.

As realized in film-works from the 1960s by LeGrice, Kren, Eatherley, Crosswaite, Warhol, Wieland, Snow, in the 1920s groundbreaking early work by Germaine Dulac (*Arabesque*, 1929) and Ester Schub's 1927 *The Fall of the Romanov Dynasty* (also the shooting script for Eisenstein's *Strike*, which she co-wrote), as well as Vertov's *Enthusiasm* and parts of *The Man With the Movie Camera*, the splice functioned as marker, as dialecticized material cut-off so that the montage could be foregrounded.[14] In many structural/materialist and post-structural/materialist

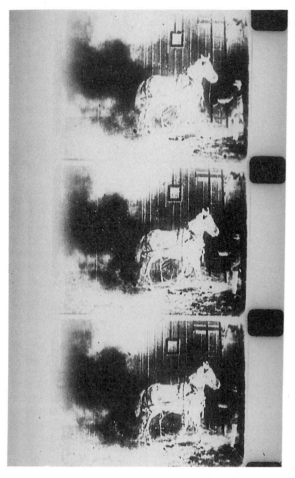

31 Malcolm LeGrice, *Berlin Horse* (1971)

films, and in the works of Lis Rhodes, Lucy Panteli, Mike
Maziere, Joanna Millet, Nicky Hamlyn, Rose Lowder, the
splice's evidence operates via the pro-filmic "content." Here
the splice, projected, is not simply another *abstract*ed *image*,
but rather a process, the holding together or not of two
disparate, or continuous, strips of film. The splice then becomes
simultaneously the interruptive and the facilitator of a form
of continuity. The splice's contradictory function, image, and

process, interruptive *and* its opposite, is produced in films which do not *codify* its suppression.

This strategy then operates in relation to other filmic strategies of each particular film. The splice in loop films could be a foregrounded cut in continuum, automatically, by the fact of the loop's recurrence as the first frame at whatever point in the repetition comes immediately after the last frame of each "loop's" material length. Yet, ineluctably, beginning and end are eventually obliterated in the film-as-projected (always co-equally depending on the contingencies of the filmed "content"). Simultaneously, this is a foregrounding antagonistic to the concept of beginning and end. Each time the last frame attached to the first repeat is projected there is a jump.

Yet there are strategies which could annihilate this materialist functioning of the loop, such as a graphic intention formulated to make a flood of light and colour beginning over and over again, a heightening of narrative pleasure, however abstracted. That is why such definitions as herein given can never be somehow adequately separated from the specific film, and the specific pro-filmic, that which is filmed. At the simplest level of structure, the loop can operate to constantly reintroduce questions of narrativity, beginning, end, and the meanings inherent filmically in those constructs. (The "opposite" strategy for a loop structure has been detailed in relation to *Condition of Illusion*, see p. 22.) Yet there are myriad possibilities for suppressing each materialist function, and graphicizing a work is but one. Various repetitions, repeated pleasurable viewings on a voyeuristic level, can heighten narrative satisfaction (due to powerful signification) without questioning any material process.

With a materialist use of splice, moment of fusion and coherence are given as a construct; disfusion similarly. Thus no *a priori* metaphor is established for which this technical convention need function as a quasi-narrative pretence.

What is also important when discussing the splice is that a film segment is marked by *two* splices, and it is simply a matter of the level of (conscious) suppression or (unconscious) repression of these. I am arguing against the notion of a solution being "*applied*" to this problematic.

Take Kren's film, *Trees in Autumn*, which is a sequence of durational segments, three seconds each, of branches, all differing, without loops or repetition. The splice mark is here an obvious cut *per se* due to the abrupt image change of each three-second strip. This is analogous to cutting on stillness, though it is not stillness in this film: trees and branches and camera *move*. Cutting on non-movement, stillness, is precisely the opposite of the first lesson in all filmschools from Prague and Warsaw to New York and Los Angeles, the National Film School and the Royal College of Art: "Always cut on movement." For conventional illusionism that is a first principle, though there are sophisticated ways of insuring narrative's seamless continuum even whilst breaking such rules. It is the *degree* of movement in a film segment that is categorized as "movement" or "stillness," as there is, paradoxically, no ontological stillness in film. The term "movement" within narrative codes means the movement of actors, cars, and so on, within a framework of action, which by definition does not allow for the subtlety let alone the precision of minimalist movement of trees, camera, frame, such as exists in the Kren film. A *complex* set of other criteria operates, even were a film ostensibly taking a "simply opposite" position from the dominant narrative codes. The "other side of the same coin" syndrome is not an applicable critique with reference to, for example, *Trees in Autumn*.

25   Filmmakers' statements

Sometimes the filmmakers' statements, since 1966 in Britain, give more than just anecdotal insight into the concerns relevant to their film-practices. Theorization attempts were never in a vacuum in relation to the film-work, though the theory is separate, the film-work is separate. Contradictions are produced in the relation between theory and practice, or, better said, between the theoretical practices of writing on film and film*making*. Filmmaking is always also theoretical.

"Since my earliest primitive film – *Castle I* – produced in a primitive and uninformed situation, my filmwork has passed through three interconnected phases. These have not been chronologically tidy, nor strictly the result of a single theoretical programme, but at the same time there have been consistent threads of conscious intent, distinguishing avant-garde film practice from that of the commercial narrative illusionist cinema. The three phases of the work broadly represent certain stages in the development of this intent. The earliest phase is that which concentrates on the material aspect of the medium as the basis of 'content', identifying celluloid, scratch, emulsion surface, sprockets, etc., and including them within the image of the film. This phase made use of various film printing devices to visibly transform small numbers of relatively short sequences of film and, as in *Little Dog for Roger* (1966), *Yes No Maybe Maybe Not* (1967), and *Berlin Horse* (1971), often concentrated on the structures.

"The next phase more consciously concentrated on establishing the screen, the screening time and space, the projection lamp and its interruption casting shadows, as the primary reality of cinema. This intent had been implicit even in the earliest films (through the device of the lightbulb actually flashing in the cinema), and periods of blank white screen in many of the other films. Though almost all the films from the start involved double-projection, usually as a method of comparing differences in treatment of the same material, in the second phase, multi-projection was combined with performance, as in *Horror Film 1*, or with deliberate movement and formatting of projectors, usually containing only loops of changing colour frames, as in *Matrix* and *Joseph's Coat*, so as to concentrate the question of materiality into the actual time/space of the projection event. This phase sought to limit or eliminate all aspects of the filmic activity not actually present with the projection event. This was not a reductionist, essentialist, purist direction, as if was often interpreted to be, but a method of establishing the primacy of the projection situation as the only material period of access available to the work by the viewer. *Pre-production*, a blank screen reading performance, indicated that however much the projection event was isolated from pre-filmic, or for that matter post-filmic, events, these were still factors which must be considered deliberately in the work.

"The next phase, which includes the most recent work, begins with *White Field Duration* and *After Leonardo* and is concerned with handling the pre-filmic (and to a lesser extent, the post-filmic) factors from the stance of the primacy of the projection event itself. From *White Field Duration* there has been a deliberate attempt to reintegrate the camera 'act' into the film procedure as a whole, in such a way that factors of reproduction, documentation, and the representation of 'incident' are dealt with as problematic, rather than unquestioningly utilized as illusionist devices. The initial step in this process involved re-filming out of the blank screen and scratched celluloid of *White Field Duration*, or the Mona Lisa reproduction taped to the blank screen during the presentation of the film.

"I do not see my work as aimed towards the expression of ideas but towards the presentation of problematic areas *as themselves* experimental content. The films *After Lumiere* and *After Manet* initiate my examination of the way in which time/space structuring of the action in the *film* and the action of the *filming* are the basis of fundamental, material content. The direction of this work has begun to allow an extension of the material basis of my film work to include enacted action between people; and to the inclusion of dialogue and narrational structure. For example, I am concerned to examine how the sequence of presentation alters the concept of the event structure of what is presented. I am concerned to extend examination of the implications of what is excluded by the frame to what is obscured by the splice. In general I would like to extend a grasp of the implications of the edit, and of time/space discontinuities, within the framework of a plausible coherence of time/space relationships.[15] In the sense of narrative or drama, these are shifted away from the narrative and drama of the illusory story to the drama of structuring time/space continuity from the material events . . . of the filmmaking and viewing" (Malcolm LeGrice, "Filmmaker's statement," *Perspectives on the English Avant Garde*, Arts Council/British Council Catalogue, 1978).[16]

The precision of this statement makes it possible to see where such a film-practice finds its purpose. An example of a particular problem for film can be elucidated with this example, and LeGrice would be the first to want a problematic. His early and constant solidarity with so many filmmakers helped to allow an advanced film culture to take place as a social practice rather than as individualization. A group of filmmakers subscribed to collective work even when the films were individually different in intent. There must be argument with LeGrice's last paragraph though, in the sense that it could displace one drama with another, as some British films following the statement do also. This theoretical miscalculation had realigned the project for a time. The narrative hold, "plausible coherence", must be seen together with its genesis from British empiricism. What this means is that whilst LeGrice was working experimentally in radical ways which were both difficult and important for British cinema, there was a reliance on the *perceptual,* on the hold of the scopic, and on the visual coherence within which meaning accrues. Though verbally articulated, this position only persisted in some of the films. LeGrice, and some of the other important filmmakers working at this time (1967–77), Annabel Nicholson, Gill Eatherley, Mike Dunford, Sally Potter, William Raban, utilized the physical presence of projectors, the projector-beam, evidence of filmmaker at the projection event, various other apparati, and so on, as part also of the projection/performance *event.* During this period, for example, at Gallery House, London, and the FilmAKTION Liverpool, there was a reliance on the empirical/physical, both of cinema technology and the filmmakers themselves as organizing coherence.

This was nevertheless distinguishable from auteurism, which those who were self-labelled "progressive critics" vehemently adhered to, viz. the writing in *Screen, Movie, Frameworks, After Image, Jump-Cut, October,* which could never take account of the specificity of any British experimental film. Except for the writings of Deke Dusinberre, A. L. Rees, and Stephen Heath, little non-auteurist writing appeared during 1967–77 other than by Co-op filmmakers/critics/polemicists/theorists.

26   Performance

The organizing tendency around the empirical real of a performance made important experimental inroads for the avant-garde through research and practice, to do with the parameters of film form (not to exclude the body). (By this time, 1974, American avant-garde film was a stultified formalism.) Nevertheless, a rerouted concern with the perceptual "truth" of an event, and, curiously, a form of documentary illusionism, were re-inserted into the proceedings. Dunford's *Still Life with Pear* (1973) and LeGrice's *After Lumiere* (1977) are examples. The theorization and film-practices against the reintegration of illusionism, narrativization, perspective, could not be somehow safe against these cultural modes. The latter found aspects of their dominance reinserted, via uncommon strategies. This difficulty though was simultaneous to advances in performance and projection events: the materiality of the referent in constant conflict with the materiality of the photochemical means of production. Causes versus effects, a necessary problematic in the British philosophical context. The problematic in those productive terms informed *most of* Eatherley's, Crosswaite's, Dunford's, and LeGrice's work as well as Raban's exceptional *2 minutes 45 seconds* (1973), and Nicholson's *Reel Time* (1973). Any difficulties enjoined were not somehow anyone's "fault," nor were there tendencies giving *credence* to dominant modes; it is simply that when ideology is assumed to be absent, it refinds its place. When a conjunction between experimental film-work and avant-garde film-work is assumed instead of being forged, ideology finds its place. You are never outside ideology.

In the same period, Marilyn Halford's work was exempt from any problem of coherence as overriding principle. In her expanded performance events, she precisely mitigated her body movements in mime to, and in necessary lack of or loss of synchronization from, the represented "her" on screen. She performed live in front of filmings of her body moving, gesturing, hands forward palms flat to screen, hands "flat" to camera. This forced the viewer not to reduce his or her perception to "perception pure and simple" but rather to the interstices of perception, that is, the contradictions imposed by the attempt at successful coherent mimesis and its endless failure. Over and over she would repeat the series of filmed gestures, live against the screen, trying, for example, to "catch up" with her own hands to a point where the represented gestures of placing her hands forward in a certain way in-film would be symmetrically "covered" by the performer (Halford) in the performance area onto the screen. The hilarity emanated from the impossibility of the performer to successfully imitate her own represented movements and gestures, to catch up. Covering them, or anticipating them, was often a split second "off" and therefore failed. This positioned the audience to at once identify with her, the body in the room, the person, and against her. This distance was wrought by self-identificatory mimesis *never at one* (i.e. never in imaginary identity) with the *performer's* synchronizations and failed attempts at synchronicity. The break between identificatory desire on the viewer's part and the actress's mimesis-attempts forced the filmic representation to

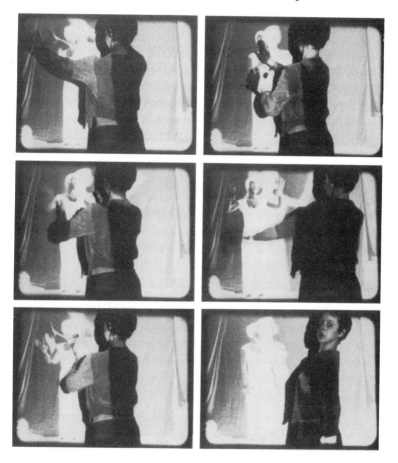

32 Marilyn Halford, *Hands Knees and Boomsa Daisy* (1974)

become co-equal with Halford's live gestural acts. The "primary" event in terms of setting the pace to be "followed" and mimed to thus took on no greater importance or truth effect, thus no *objectification*, or making an object, of the "other." All blatantly an act, merely a necessary structure for the live imitation, of what was in any case shown as an imitation on film in the first place, of Halford. The image, and the image of an image, the former trying to catch up with the latter. The comic tradition of British music-hall was no further from this than the history of cinema and philosophico-aesthetic enquiry.

Problems with film and "expanded" performance are articulated by Gill Eatherley, whose own work at the time (1970–4) played an important part. The moments to watch are those that realize already in 1973 the questions of the subjectivity of the filmmaker, a subjectivity with no implication of authorship. Eatherley also recognizes that the questions must pertain to the filming and viewing subject positioned in a contradictory historical locus. Her film performance and multi-screen works produced a fractured subjectivity in constant conflict with social meaning(s). Film-work as historical (not historicizing) space and time, a common factor in the works discussed.

"Things started with a definite movement away from painting to some mini-trials with a stills camera and its time exposure device. Produced static recordings of light bulb traces in a black space: with two results – one, unsatisfactory; two, began working with film. The attitudes behind the early popcorn movies can explain themselves – a travelling difference, trajectory, and film concern, up to the making of *Meanwhile* (1971), my film-and-light film, as part of "Light Occupations." My first dealings on film involved preoccupations with processes of editing, recorded rhythms and energies, and subsequent relationships between elements, plus some colour printing – *Hand Grenade*. Then in *Deck* (1972) the basic format alights from a re-filming, breaking down the screen size, pulse, shape, and transformation. *Pan Film* and *Shot Spread* are derived more directly from straight camera/eye observations, topology of film and its limitations. *Shot Spread* has a strict cutting score between the three screens, shifting the "image" from left to right. Now, basic concerns with film syntax have been interrelated with the audience/film presentation-situation. For although the word

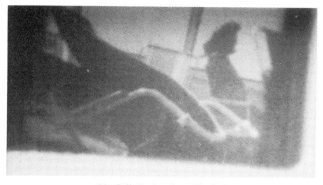

33 Gill Eatherley, *Deck* (1972)

"expanded" cinema has also been used for the open/gallery size/multiscreen presentation of film, this "expansion" (could still but) has not *yet* proved satisfactory – for my own work anyway. Whether you are dealing with a single postcard size screen or six ten-foot screens, the problems are basically the same – to try to establish a more positively dialectical relationship with the audience. I am concerned (like many others) with this balance between the audience and the film – and the noetic problem involved. There have been many struggles with projection ideas, which are impossible to realize, due to lack of situations outside the conventional cinema in London. . . . I would like to be able to do a little more than just be cinematically

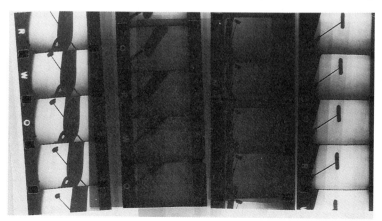

34 Gill Eatherley, *Aperture Sweep* (1973)

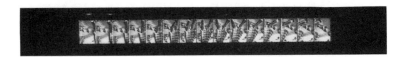

35 Gill Eatherley, *4 Screen Film*

squatting – while the films disappear, to be shown in someone's filmclub at the other end of the country – and any reaction from an audience, and the film's physical reality, is projected miles away from me. The filmmakers' own direct awareness of the presentation of the work and the audience are equally important to the film as its own emulsion. Like we sometimes feel 'the axeman has a foot in the door to our heads' the viewer might think 'the filmmaker has a film in the gate of their head' " (Gill Eatherley, "Filmmaker's statement," "The Avant Garde" exhibition, Gallery House, London, 1972).

When Eatherley stopped making films, she was one of the core group at the London Film Co-op who found no way out of certain cinematic dilemmas. The toll taken in avant-garde movements is always distressing; those who are no longer producing helped define the way we all saw the problematics of cinema in the first place. Equally important was the solidarity one received in that group; without that the whole core group of 1966–74 would have stopped working. As it is, Eatherley, Crosswaite, Hammond, Du Cane, Potter, Dunford, found it impossible to go on in this area. The considerable power, beauty, and quantity of, and the issues raised through, the early works are still of extreme importance to film and art nearly two decades later.

27 Film as material

The assertion of "film as material" is predicated upon representation, inasmuch as "pure" empty acetate running through the projector-gate without image, for example, merely sets off another level of associations. These can be abstract, or not. But they are, when instigated by such a device, no more materialist or anti-illusionist than any other associations. Thus the film event is by no means necessarily demystified. "Empty screen" is no less significatory than "carefree smile" or "murderous chase." There are myriad possibilities for co-optation and integration of filmic procedures into the repertoire of meaning. The persistent attempt to misunderstand this has led to blind alleys for attempted analytical criticism of experimental film these last twenty years, and also for the works themselves at times. Film must be constructed in such a way that it does not fall into the "myriad possibilities of meaning." This necessitates a theoretical stance which understands the concrete consequences of the notion of abstraction and the abstract. Abstract work, so-called, can (but does not have to) be as full of the associative, identificatory pull, narrativizational mechanisms, as anything else, as there is no ontology.

Peter Kubelka's *Arnulf Rainer* (1966, Austria) "is a montage of black and white leader, with white sound (a mixture of all audible frequencies)" (P. Adams Sitney, *Visionary Film*, Oxford University Press, New York, 1974, p. 335). Kubelka himself argues that the strongest collisions are between frames, that it is not the shots which collide but "the last frame of one and the first frame of the other" (ibid.). Such a flicker film does not materially present pure cinema. Rather, it is again another means towards a melodic end, derivative of serial music structures, and, for the filmmaker, "it is an evocation of the dawn, of day and night, of thunder and lightning" (ibid.). The abstract can be full of the associative, narrativizational, but the reverse is not the case. The narrativizational, identificatory story film can not empty out its significations. If it could, it could do so only through a philosophical sleight-of-hand: to reproduce a series of narrative spaces and times, actions, personae, psychologies, then empty them, would be to paradoxically deny the "them" on which the operation is based. Theorizable or not, in the material praxis of film it would be concretely impossible because of cultural cinematic and extra-cinematic determinate meanings adhering. These meanings adhere to representations and images. Every image, in film and out, is an image of an image, that is, a representation. In other words, it is always already a reproduced and held cultural convention: positioned historically, sexually, economically.

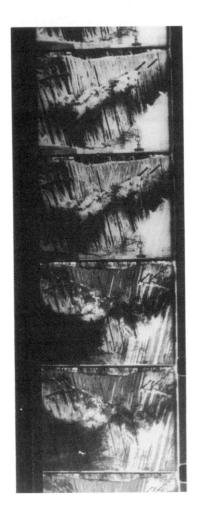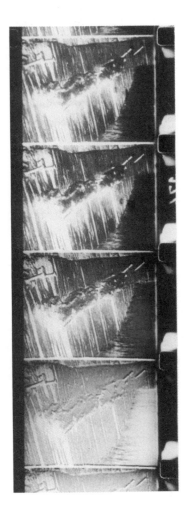

36(a) Malcolm LeGrice, *Yes No Maybe Maybe Not* (1967)

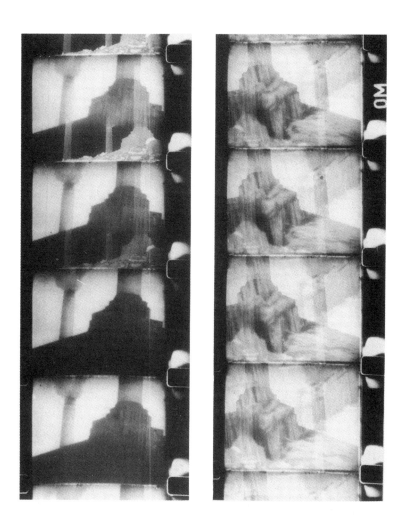

36(b) Malcolm LeGrice, *Yes No Maybe Maybe Not* (1967)

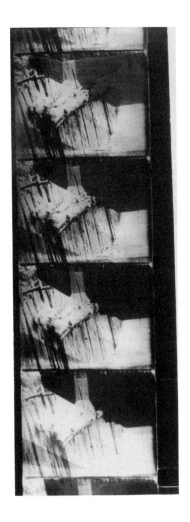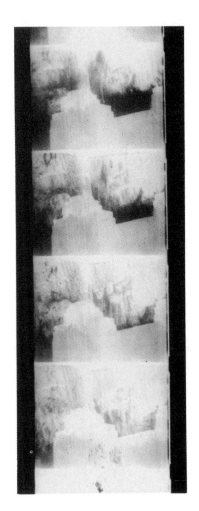

36(c) Malcolm LeGrice, *Yes No Maybe Maybe Not* (1967)

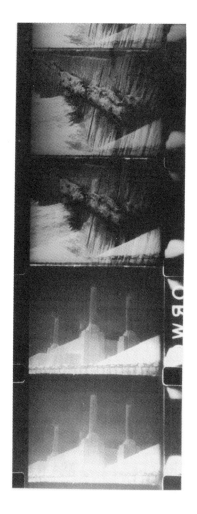 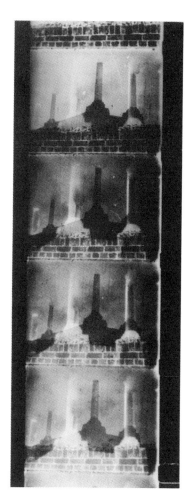

36(d) Malcolm LeGrice, *Yes No Maybe Maybe Not* (1967)

An example of anti-narrative work that does *not* reproduce "myriad possibilities" for the integration of narrative and identity is LeGrice's *Yes No Maybe Maybe Not* (1967). The viewer's conscious and unconscious mechanisms within the film-as-projected's duration makes for dialectical material. Such film can utilize the rubric *Realist* precisely because it functions to *unplace* the spectator for the film's duration, to place him/her in a radical stance – a new "spectator," a new "subject." Realism of another kind. How is this new constructed? A viewer *not* "in-the-know."

There are two basic sequences in *Yes No Maybe Maybe Not*. An image of water splashing against a wall or barrier, and a long shot of Battersea power station, with its huge smokestacks, smoke rising out of them. The strategy includes elements of chance in editing. The film "starts" with a negative image of water superimposed upon the image-positive. Then we see Battersea power station superimposed upon itself (again negative on positive filmstock). *Then* we come to variations of the power station through a change in synchronization, the negative is held back about four frames, and the synch is lost, creating a space between negative and positive. Following this, the water is superimposed upon the Battersea power station, to give us a triple layer of movement. The space between two equal opposite images that are several frames out of synch makes for the effect of bas-relief; also, the separation of two images, one negative, one postitive, makes for a line-determined space of grey that varies in shape and tone according to the change of synchronization (moving the negative another five, six, seven, eight frames ahead of the positive). The interplay of *same* images creates a dialectic, which becomes more complex via the viewer.

The further two same images go out of synch, the larger the grey in-between shape becomes. From *space* "between" we produce "image." It is nothing. As this new image is the product of the space usually considered a negative space, formed by the separation of two (filmstock negative and filmstock positive) image-layers, one cannot immediately grasp hold of the precise situation when watching it. To add to this, the second image of Battersea power station involves itself to the same triple extent. The intermittent negative shapes formed are defined by line. The image of foreground and background becomes reversed, and through the abstraction process we lose sight of three-dimensional space representation. This reversal of foreground/background through the varying tones of grey, and intermittent spaces created, functions somewhat like high contrast silhouette images wherein one cannot tell which of the two shapes predominates, the black or white cutout. That is what "defined by line" is meant to mean. As we focus on a specific spatial aspect of a frame, or, more correctly, series of frames (as it is twenty-four frames per second) we become aware of the process of image-separation. We react to *this*. The process-viewing itself is the content of this film. This becomes apparent, i.e. a conscious reflexivity is instanced, as well as the unconscious processes of relation of the spectator to the seen but unknown, the supposedly apprehendable unapprehendable.

The film consists primarily of a thirty-foot (fifty-second) sequence of the water, and a twenty-five-foot sequence of Battersea power station. After LeGrice, who printed the film himself, came to the end of each section, he would start over with the same piece of material. The images themselves are not found images. They were filmed by LeGrice to be used for this film; but they do not immediately look as if they were definitely *not* found footage. This history of cinema has its codings for what "looks" like found footage, often fairly grey documentary shots of this or that, out-takes from one of an endless series of documentaries. The second aspect of the footage not giving itself as definitely *not* found footage is that the images are not seemingly chosen images that serve a specific purpose of *meaning prior to the film*. That is, their "content" is denotative, descriptive, to the point of *not* forcing interferences of assumed connotative meaning other than of supposedly neutral docu-mentation. This assumption is already, though, based on the way these specific shots are used in *this* film. These shots used in a thriller would, as separable shots "prior" to the film, seem to have precisely those meanings loaded into their content that the later montage gives them.

Thus, it is never a matter of contextless footage ahistorically containing an essence of meaning. The context is inseparable. The play of the horizontal waves crashing repeatedly against the barrier, the Battersea power station inseparably printed through, results in condensation, signifiers overlapping, images condensed to produce "more," yet not giving the result as some reversible conglomerate which could be reduced to its parts. The transformations of meaning take place through this condensation-process. The repetitions in this film point to an obsessiveness which effects through the viewer a start/stop/start syndrome disallowing closure at any moment, and resisting the viewer's resistances to its compulsions. The viewer is not made to feel he/she knows, is not in and at one with a representation. There is thus no reality that is produced as the object for this subject "I."

When the waves hit the barrier again and again, with varying degrees of intermittent shape formed by the negative/positive image, we are led to studiously *see* each nuance of change. The mechanics of the nuance betray less a humanistic "hand touch" sensibility (however much that may have been part of the process) or artistic presence-in-absence; rather, material differences of effect. The loop effect, which can never be ascertained with certainty, makes for a gap in our knowledge: we do not know, and we know we do not know, whether the wave-loop is a repeat of the previous montage segment. Is it similar or is it the same? The *it* recedes from status as document and referent and putative signifieds, as the materiality of the film-loop endures. Illusionistic three-dimensional space, photochemically reproduced, and two dimensional "abstract" space, form the film image. Yet *this* film makes sophisticated use of both and disallows a separability of *concept* from the *concrete*. It is precisely by not letting "the abstract" become ahistorical (something *other*) that this film remains part of the cinematic social institution and its concerns. The abstract does not separate from the reproductions dealt with, from, more precisely, *the fact that they are reproductions of concrete material reality, attempted representations*. The opposite problem, not of the abstract but of positivizing a three dimensional representation, separating it from the abstract and thus holding onto the three dimensional illusion as if that were cinema pure and simple, would be *to separate the reproductions from filmic material i.e. from concrete abstract reality*. Thus both the abstract and the represented real are concrete, and (the concept of) materialist film theorizes the inseparability of the two in practice (i.e. they are still "two" not "one").

Dialectical materialism: the dynamic interconnectedness of things and concepts. Or rather, "the theory of reality affirming the continuous transformation of matter, and the dynamic interconnectedness of things and concepts, and implying social transformation through socialism toward a classless society, which was advanced by Marx and Engels and adopted as official Soviet philosophy" (*Webster's Collegiate Dictionary*, 1971).

The obsessive repetition of question/answer dialectic is shown as part of the intention of the title (of the author?!). That intention and "result" are separate does not mean we must avoid either. It is though not to read out what was put in, as if the film were a transparent vehicle for communication. It is, rather, to see that the contexting via the verbal, within which so much meaning (some say all) exists as "symbolic" in our culture, is important. Simply that. This thought process, the internalized dialectic with the "self," the posing of question and anti-question towards maybe-not, disallowing thereby the jigsaw-puzzle aspect of questioning, which both high art and high Hollywood cinema attempts, is a preoccupation for this film via the context of its title and the mechanisms of its production process, as film. The relations must still be constructed through an anti-psychoanalytic spectation and its histories within cinema culture. The real is problematized. A reproduction is not held into a representation.[17] "For us, the 'real' is not a *theoretical slogan*; the real is the real object that exists independently of its knowledge – but which can only be defined by its knowledge" (Althusser, *For Marx*, transl. Ben Brewster, Allen Lane, The Penguin Press, London, 1969, p. 246). Any relation to the real and its transformations in this film *Yes No Maybe Maybe Not* is to that whereas in dominant cinema it is to precisely not that.

The "other" space created by the one, roll A, and the other, roll B, is a grey other space as described, the filmstock neither negative nor positive . Imagery, or "the shots", are the effect of a (film-)process. That film, or impossible representation, is a determinate effect of a labour process, materialist. Image functions as what is left, residue. This unfulfillment without the illusion of fulfillment is that of Beckett, Stein, Warhol, Delphy, rather than a quasi-religious paternity of Joyce, Elliot, Brakhage, Kristeva.[18] (See original form of the essay on *Yes No Maybe Maybe Not* for what were then just the beginnings of a materialist theorization in *Ark: The Journal of the Royal College of Art*, London, Spring, 1970).[19]

28   Cinema verité

"Cinema verité is posited on the ability of the camera to record meaningful events, these events having structured themselves so that the camera can claim and recall their veracity. One does not have to assume that the events filmed have this sort of veracity, distinct from their presence in cinema – some examples make it perfectly obvious that what is being shown does not in a mystical sense pre-exist the cinema that produced it – the spaces shown, we are then informed, are there because of their place in the film. As in direct looks at the camera (Leaud in Godard, for example) moments are presented that show the role of the pro-filmic as literally 'for the film' which displays them (Godard) rather than as pre-cinematic with the cinema present as historical accident (cinema verité)" (A. L. Rees, "Conditions of illusionism," *Screen*, vol. 18, no. 3, 1977).

The main point is not to limit this idea to anything approaching the direct *look back* at the filmmaker/audience, as that can simply enlarge the imaginary world alluded to, but to not find the *look* at all. The "look", whether "to" the viewer or "at" someone in the document or fiction, is a constituting basis for conventional realisms. Literalness must be produced without illusionist description. Thus, in the example of *Yes No Maybe Maybe Not*, the specificity of the structure is articulated *through* cinematic construction and not through (imagined or real) literary content. Thus *not* through diegesis, which would incorporate as content the *veracity of* filmic construction itself. The question of the content's veracity is thus a red herring, sidestepping the problematic and reintegrating, through the back door as it were, the omniscient narrator, or voice of truth, or evidence, whilst ostensibly operating against the crude ideology of cinema verité.

29   Audience numbers and sex

Mick Eaton writes in "The avant garde and narrative": "Gidal writes 'The dialectic of the film is established in that space of tension between materialist flatness, grain, light, movement, and the supposed real reality that is represented.' Again I feel that the danger of a structural/materialist aesthetic lies in placing too great an emphasis on the former terms without adequately coming to terms with the latter. If this course is adopted it can certainly only lead to a stifling of that very dialectic whose terms are obviously so vital in any interventionist practice. In fact, a concentration in film practice on substance over signification can lead to a retreat, not only from editing, but also from performance, verbal language, and writing. We have to ask ourselves how politically viable at the present time is a cinema which rejects non-cinematic codes? The issue of performance is not as trivial as it may appear. Although 'acting' as a representational code is, of course, non-cinematic, it has been fused with cinematic codes since the earliest days of cinema and the transparency and seeming inevitability of this fusion will not be ruptured by denying this history. . . . It seems dangerous to proscribe a film practice which does attempt to deal dialectically with the processes of performance if only because in the most naive and sociologistic sense this mechanism of identification is one of the most crucial means by which cinemas are filled. To reject this as an issue not pertinent to the matter of film seems to indicate not only an unwillingness to intervene in what, for a large number of cinema-goers is the very matter of film – i.e. stories, characters, etc. – but also the impossibility of any kind of Brechtian practice in which what is represented enters into a dialectic with the way in which it is represented. . . . I am . . . merely suggesting that perhaps it is not necessary for the structural/materialist film-maker to reject dealing with performance, or indeed other non-cinematic codes, in advance" (Mick Eaton, "The avant garde and narrative," *Screen*, Summer 1978, p. 133). Sally Potter (*Thriller*, 1978) faltered on that idea. "For *The Gold Diggers* (1983) she thought she'd get a new, different, and big audience. I had to finally explain to her that no distributor was going to put up over £100,000 to get *The Gold Diggers* distributed, that is, £100,000 above its £200,000 costs (from Channel 4 and the BFI). No one can understand what's going on in the film! It's not experimental but it is confusing! No one is going to put up the £100,000 that would be needed to get it to different venues from the usual ones. Yet such venues would be necessary to recoup costs! I like the film, but there's no audience for it." This response to a film which was made as "popularist" shows the pitfalls of taking, with all good intentions, a condescending and paternalistic view of cinema-goers, as Eaton and Potter do. It leads to what Lenin called objective opportunism. There is no in-built elitism adhering to experimental materialist work. Current forms of cultural domination, ideological and economic, must be smashed. The alternative is opportunism becoming the only possibility for those independent filmmakers and critics who disavow a materialist avant-garde. Breaks in the system allow some work to be done which questions the premises of representation. Fundamental to the above remains the question of to what degree a massive change in public structures of representing *must* be instituted for a radical change to take place; that is, for a change in film, in the social meanings and individual positions produced through film.

Jacqueline Rose has written: "On the one hand, there is (with structural/materialist film) the discussion as to types of object represented. This raises, for example, the whole question of the relative potency of images . . . the avoidance of the socially coded objects of fetishism, the refusal to produce and reproduce film images of women and hence the refusal to use images of women or men. With this, the symptomatic duality that this then imposes: against anthropomorphic identification[20] through the narrative relations of human figures, which means images of men or women, and, also, the inevitable stressed addition to the general rule, against images of women, specifically, and whether in or out of conventional narrative (the point of Laura Mulvey's emphases in her essay "Visual pleasure and narrative cinema," that the image of the woman is the best way of stopping narrative flow *without* trouble, unpleasure). At one level, this position is clear, if pessimistic: the objects to be subjected to the film process should not be the culturally received objects of fetishism and censor. The fact that it is the image of the woman that here causes the split in the theory, forcing the filmmaking activity to think itself on two fronts, foregrounds this very problem of women and representation" (Jacqueline Rose, "Problems in current theory" *The Cinematic Apparatus*, Macmillan, London, 1981; St Martins Press, New York, 1986, p. 180, reprinted in Rose's *Sexuality in the Field of Vision*, Verso-NLB, London, 1986). Rose argues further: "A confusion at the level of sexuality brings with it a disturbance of the visual field. . . . There can be no work on the image, no challenge to its power of illusion and address, which does not simultaneously challenge the fact of sexual difference. . . . As if Freud found the aptest analogy for the problem of our identity as human subjects in failures of vision. . . . Something which can only come into focus now by blurring the field of representation where our normal forms of self-recognition take place. . . .

"The unconscious reveals that the normal divisions of language and sexuality obey the dictates of an arbitrary law and undermine the very possibility of reference for the subject since the 'I' can no longer be seen to correspond to some pre-given and permanent identity of psychosexual life. The problem of psychic identity is therefore immanent to the problem of the sign. . . . The image (therefore) submits to the sexual reference, but only insofar as reference itself is questioned by the work of the image" (Rose, "Sexuality in the field of vision," in the book of the same name, op.cit.).

The theoretical problematic so precisely elucidated above could (but does not have to) get stuck in the notion that some form of sexual representation, an *object*, is necessary to problematize the sexual positioning of the viewer-subject, the "I". At the same time critiques must be formulated *against* "the more recent practice of appropriating artistic and photographic images in order to undermine their previous status" (Mike O'Pray, "Movies, mania, and masculinity," *Screen*, 1983, pp. 63–70). The latter being another form of deconstruction. If one theorizes the image, the referent, as culturally/politically

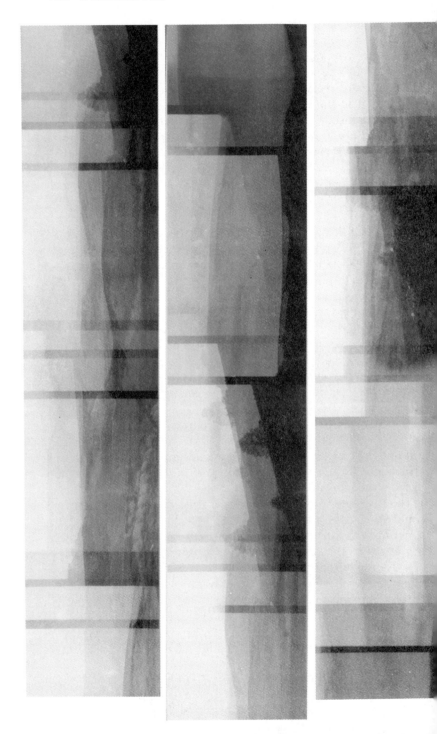

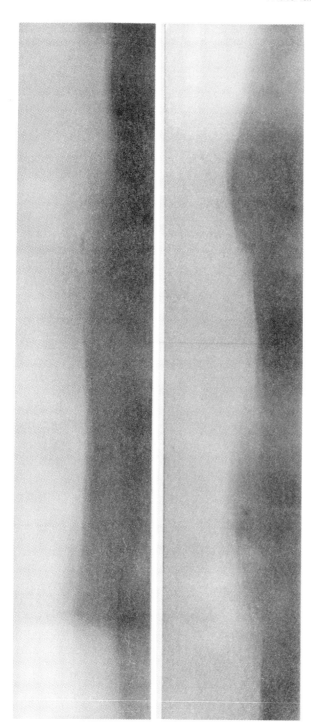

37 Joanna Millet, *Views from Ilford Hill* (1983)

overdetermined in the case of sexual representation, then there is no way to fully represent the female or male body, and/or sexuality, whilst at the same time somehow "blurring the field of representation," unless that blurring is to leave the field of representation and "our normal forms of self-recognition" intact. In order, thus, not to fall into an idealist utopia, or a repressed "solving" of the problematic in a way which reinstates its solidity as dominant form, the film-work must either absent sexual representation altogether, at this historical juncture, or minimize it to such an extent that recognizability is always questioned/questionable already at the perceptual (as well as unconscious) levels. That then can engage with dominant forms, memories, and knowledge of sexual representation, and problematize/radicalize *or make impossible* attempted identities. "Men have sex with their image of a woman. Escalating explicitness, 'exceeding the bounds of candour', is the aesthetic of pornography not because the materials depict objectified sex but because they create the experience of a sexuality which is itself objectified" (Catharine MacKinnon, "Not a moral issue," *Yale Law Review*, vol. 2, no. 291, 1984, p. 3289). To which Lisa Cartwright states: "This explains Baudrillard's prescriptive for heightened reproduction and proliferation of objectified sexuality," in patriarchy's interests of reiterating (via fetish (replacement of one's own, not the other's, lack) and metaphor) maleness and its organized force. Thus the strategy of pastiche, irony, and the simulacra are of use only in so far as power and its effects are thereby solidified via said fetish and metaphor. Phallocracy's (and the male's) power is endless impotence endlessly repressed. "The new (American) art's" immediate popularity is also the result thereof (neo-geo/neo-conceptualism/etc.).

"Triumph in phantasy equally achieves the effect of denying dependence whilst at the same time by that very control acceding to the dependence denied, – while also denying any feelings of value characteristically ascribed to the mother and breast. Phantasies involving contempt for the object denies the object's power to cause experiences of loss and guilt. This triad of triumph, control, and contempt also justifies attacks on the objects, ensuing in even severer feelings of loss and guilt, and so demanding more manic defence and so on. There seems

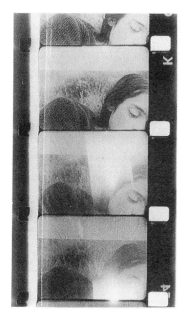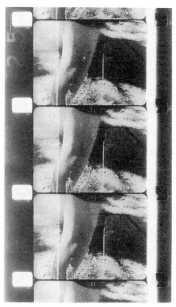

38 Mike Maziere, *Image Moment*, two-screen (1985)

little doubt that the representation of women in our culture
is very often determined by such phantasies. (On the other
hand) in Nicky Hamlyn's *Not to See Again* (1980) the abstract
quality (never total, for the objects are always recognizable as
objects) helps Hamlyn to negotiate sexual imagery as it occurs
in the film by rendering those images relatively abstract and
on a par almost with other objects depicted. Close-up, colour,
shape, mass, and texture subvert the meaning of the object,
also rendering the naked body (male and female . . . [in]
awareness of film as process and material and the image itself
as meaning, constructed in that process) almost abstract. The
effect, of course, is to drain the image of its conventional sexual
meanings and associations (with pornography, for instance)
and instead neutralize it almost – *almost*, for what remains is
a representation of sexuality which is not privileged in either
an idealized way or an attacking aggressive mode. It is simply
there as an area of colour, light, movement, shape, texture
– almost (again) the representation of the object shed of its

conventional associations. . . . Here, objects and bodies are not simply psychologistic or dramatic means to resolution, and may develop without reduction to the glossy, or pornographic, and the narrative device" (O'Pray, op.cit.). This would be the attempt at the post-structural/materialist necessity taken to the point of insistent sexual reference, rather than the reference lacking sexuality. Other strategies are taken by Lis Rhodes in *Light Reading* (1978), Joanna Millet in *Views from Ilford Hill* (1983), Mike Maziere in *Colour Work* (1982), Lucy Panteli in *Motion Picture* (1980) and *Photo Play* (1984), Josef Robakowski in *From a Window* (1986), W. and B. Hein in their work 1968–74 and the Aleinikov brothers of Moscow's Ciné-Phantom since 1986, Yann Beauvais in *Void* (1986), Coredelia Swann in *Phantoms* (1986), Carole Enahoro in *Oyinbo Pepper* (1986), Bill Brand in *Coalfields* (1984), Black Audio Film Collective's and Sankofa's work, Anna Thew's *Hilda was a Good-Looker* (1985), etc.

My films including *Close Up* (1983), *Denials* (1985), and *Guilt* (1988) have also been attempts at other strategies.

30   Rose Lowder's *Composed Recurrence* (1981)

Rose Lowder's *Composed Recurrence* is analysed by radical feminist film theorist Lisa Cartwright: "*Retour d'un Repère Composé (Composed Recurrence)* is a film made by Rose Lowder in France in 1982. The film is composed of a 2 3/4 minute long negative – a shot of a branch before water printed eight times singly, eight times superimposed onto a second print, out of phase (i.e. so that the images don't perfectly match or superimpose on each other) and eight times printed as a triple super-imposition, again out of phase(s). The structure is repeated every 2 1/2 seconds (that is, the initial 2 3/4 minutes mentioned are made up of a segment 2 1/2 seconds long, repeated mechanically) using a verse form called a *pantoun*, as a device for organizing the sections into units. Beginning by speaking of what *Retour* is *not* may not be the most useful way of speaking of the film. The need to speak in the terms of "like" films, however, has to be addressed before going on to the particular ways in which the film functions differently from other experimental film.

"The dominance of reductive criticisms and analyses of experimental films has led to a near-contempt for any attempt towards speaking about current experimental film in other than metaphysical terms. With few exceptions, such films have been talked into obscurity before any *real* history could develop – one which takes into account the specifics of film, its material, and the differences between the films produced. In speaking of the problem of context, Rose Lowder writes 'It would be a mistake to see this work as starting on similar premises to that of all films using systematic approaches. . . .' One area of experimental filmmaking given currency lately is that of the formalist fratriarch of American structural filmmaking. This particular area is safe ground, politically neutral in that their filmic 'discoveries' took place last decade. A shared context being unavoidable, there being no getting away from film in making films, *Retour d'un Repère Composé* can easily be placed into this tradition. In doing so, however, the way in which Lowder's film stands in opposition to American structural film is overlooked.

"The latter films provide a clear *picture* of what the film in question here is *not*. Formal films of the seventies are marked by the sentiment that experimentation in film is *fully realized* possibility, its end repeated in ironic filmic lamentations over the frustrating impossibility of (hence depiction of a frustrated need for) a use of film to reveal. These filmic illustrations take on a certain *familiarity* among themselves, relating back in a less immediate way to the patriarch, narrative film, ultimate knowledge of the common object sought/lost.

"In short there is nothing left for *these* filmmakers to say.

"In watching *Retour d'un Repère Composé* what becomes apparent is that nothing is familiar, nothing is revealed. The initial image lasts throughout the film but undergoes continual transformation. The *obvious* nature of that image being as before stated a branch-in-front-of-water at once and continually broken by the continual movement of the screen, continual seeming movement based on the staccato superimpositions previously described.

"What kind of film is it? It is an avant-garde, experimental, and materialist feminist film. It is rigorous in that it works in

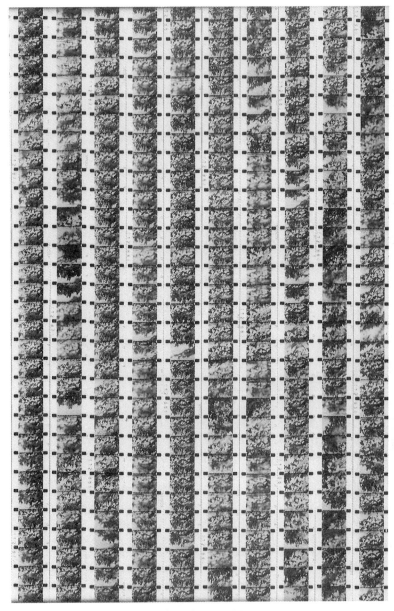

39 Rose Lowder, *Composed Recurrence* (1981)

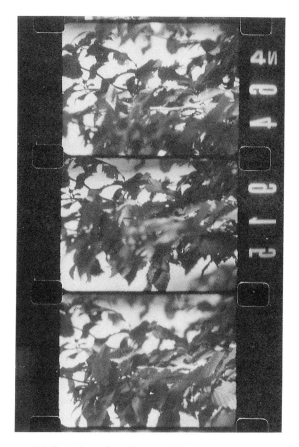

40 Rose Lowder, *Composed Recurrence* (1981)

a total way against the repositioning of meaning, with its basis in sexual division, at every level. It works against the meaning of 'good' movie-making at the level of the most 'neutral' concept of representation, and the most 'technical' concepts of film production – levels which are usually 'forgotten.' What this 'forgetting' means for avant-garde film is that it provides a point – the main point – at which relations of sexual division can be re-established, unnoticed. It proceeds from the most banal rules for 'good' movie-making by challenging the 'logical' connection between an image and the object which that image represents. The initial recognition (of images *of* leaves *as* leaves) is not assumed, but is shown as an impossible assumption. Representation is revealed as a process which can *not* work, cannot reproduce the real. This fundamental material impossibility is possible only within the given logic, the logic based on sexual division. It is this 'logic' which is the logic of 'good' movie-making. Such terms and processes at once provide the basis for the real and are materially impossible. It is materially impossible, for instance, that men/women relationships *could* be reproduced through images; notwithstanding, it is inevitably the primary task of 'good' movies to do just that – to extend the idealist, dominant ideology of sexual division as reality itself, by creating a 'logical' framework based on a material impossibility. This idealism is the methodology of male dominance, it is how it reproduces itself.

"It is incompatible with the fundamental idealism of the logic of 'good' movie-making to allow for a materialist feminist method as a material possibility. Doing this would cause a revolution in knowledge which might reveal the material impossibility of the tenets of this logic! This is exactly why, in every field, it is materialist feminist work which is *not* acknowledged, not dealt with in depth, is ignored and cannot proceed to extend its analysis, its work. Hence *Retour d'un Repère Composé's* status as 'the most rigorous film of its kind' *and* as ignored.

"The development of the film leads to no ultimate 'knowledge' of image, of *this* image, but to a present knowledge of it being *not a likeness but continually anew*. Within the film nothing is sought nor is anything held. Both the rhythm structure and the 'original' composition are indiscernable as such, as 'form', in the fragmentation and dislocation of the unity of the screen. Any understanding of the film as *composed* is impossible. The repetition, rather than providing a chance to see more clearly, leads to 'less and less.' *The longer one watches the less one ultimately knows.* The order of the familiar is shattered in not a denial of what *was* (then) but in a constant now.

"*Retour* is a materialist film which radically breaks from the metaphysics of structural filmmaking which preceded it. The film presents only the beginning of what still remains to be discovered in film" (Lisa Cartwright, typescript, March 1983, and from "The front line and the rear guard," *Screen*, November 1984, pp. 63–4).

No stare is possible in this film. There is absence, of the body, and of the body of language. Nervousness at the body's absence is the loss of the *reassurance*-of the body. It is the male loss of the body of *power*. No body for the being needed and needing to be needed to be reassured: by not functioning within the realm of possibility of metaphor, a film-work is also separated from the possibilities of being a "pure" film-object, "refusing to be undermined in its autonomy by being object or even process-object" (Malcolm LeGrice, "Some recent thoughts on film," *Millenium Film Journal*, no. 13 (winter 1983), pp. 19–31).

What we are given in *Composed Recurrence* are dialectical representations. These give no power to *either* sex of spectator; thus any imaginary self-identification is fragmented at best. Such a realism is loss. And those with institutionalized power have that to lose. This male loss is here in a regime, cinema, that ordinarily functions to solidify power and authority. Film as body as embodiment is radically opposed to film as de-anthropomorphized process. And "text" must not become euphemism for body; the literal against metaphor is the needed politic.

The loss of the body, the nervousness at the body's absence, functions differently for the viewer/woman than for the viewer/man. But equally, fear *of* the body is rejected by such usages of loss; fear induced by the representation and loss of the body is a different register of "desire" for the viewer than fear not induced by the representation and loss of the body. All the more so as the body being the "site" of power is currently a peculiarly male phantasy and truth. (Paradoxically(?) women spend much more body-power in daily work than men with their body phantasies/realities would dream of. That is the cause of phantasy, the fetish replacement precisely of what is feared both as *present* (supposed difference) and as *loss*. Women cannot be somehow outside the series of positions that patriarchy subjects them to; but the operation that situates the viewer-as-male produces a repression of women and women's struggles, histories, positions. "Difference" is never outside of ideology). The positioning of the female viewer by films which represent, or are metaphors for, the body (the fetish object) is radically opposite to the positioning of the female viewer through films which do not. The unidentifiable (in both senses) viewer is subject/object through a radically materialist film such as *Composed Recurrence*. Once "the subject" and "the object" as separable identities held to a body, or its metaphors, no longer function, a different cathexis is produced, that of process itself. The radicalization of representation is the political radicalization of the subject-in-its-history; the above is a social process, subjecting/objecting.

Catharine MacKinnon states: "They represent us very badly out there, do they not? Some days I wish they would just stop representing me, us, period. Just stop" (Lisa Cartwright and Abigail Norman, "Interview with Catharine MacKinnon," New York City, November 1984, pt I, p. 4, unpublished). She continues: "But the question is, if you have a woman and a man making sex with each other, given the place of sexuality in the subordination of women, can what you have be socially and politically equal? Is the woman seen as *as* equal as the man by the viewer? . . . You also have lookedatness happening. I don't know what 'female gaze' means, unless it means whatever a biological female does. It doesn't make it ours. Maybe it's that glazed look, looking back at the camera. The look of a woman having her picture taken, being watched looking female. It's how we are told to look when we are being looked at. To get real empirical about it, the feminine is what it is" (ibid., pt II, p. 6).

"The women doing that are the 'prosex' anti-antipornography women who are making all the 'positive' representations, going around saying they're rediscovering our sexuality which is really the same sexuality that we've been taught as ours all our lives. They're representing the same old thing as something new by simply calling it something different, or by understanding 'ours' as somehow unconditional, free. That is hopeless. On the other hand, the feminists who are challenging forms of representation without attempting directly to develop new forms and images – feminists working against representation – may proceed negatively, but this is in no way a hopeless project. To call that hopeless would be like saying that because pornography is irredeemable – in that there is no way to use it and it must be done away with – the position against it is one of hoplessness, a dead end. In both cases it's not a matter of lacking hope in one's own or other women's work, but a matter of recognizing the hopelessness in particular sexist processes that are, for women, bankrupt. That kind of hopelessness is empowering. Just as the process by which pornography works is hopeless for women and is therefore worked against, so might the process by which representation works be hopeless. And they are not unrelated. The latter is hopeless but that isn't therefore a hopeless situation for women. A position against representation isn't a position of hopelessness" (Lisa Cartwright, ibid., pp. 8 and 9).

The difficulties in writing about such work as Rose Lowder's *Composed Recurrence* are not new. Ben Brewster, who can articulate with precision the problems of Marx's notion of capital in relation both to fetishism and to Althusser's problematizing of such long ago readily admitted the problems involved in writing about the signifier in film: "It's almost impossible to write about films like *Wavelength* or *Room Film 1973* and others, because their work is with the signifier. It's almost impossible to state something about that process . . . there's no language for it" (Ben Brewster, Edinburgh Film Festival, August 1976). The hesitancy in some of the writing in this book attests to this difficulty.

31   Kurt Kren's *TV* (1966)

TV (1966) is made up of five shots, maximum four seconds each, repeated in various orders.[21] No schema can be read off of this due to the seemingly random succession, and repetition, of shots. Expectancy can never be fulfilled as to what follows or what would logically come before any of the five shots. Whether or not an arithmetic "system" preceded the making becomes irrelevant. It is only during, and some time after, the viewing(s) that the fact of its being made up of five shots becomes apparent, and even this is not as to the number "five" but as to the fact of a specifiable, even if uncountable, number of (finite) sequences being variously repeated. Thus even the fact of a determinate number of repeats cannot, whilst the film is being viewed, be reduced to a mechanization which would state the number "five" or would even certify an approximation. Additionally, black leader intervenes, taking equal power to

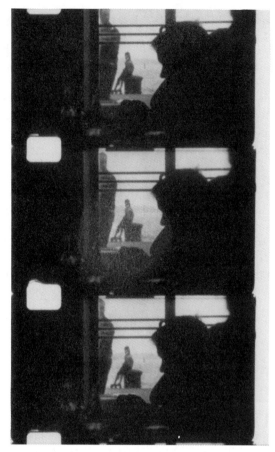

41 Kurt Kren, *TV* (1966)

the "content"-shots. Whether the black leader is interruption or simply another kind of sequence remains a question which interferes productively with the possibility of (ac)counting.

The reading into deep space, possible when the shots are viewed frozen on an editing table, is impossible when viewing the projected film, due to the speed of movement, and the quick passing of each shot-length (each is no longer than four seconds!). Thus the shot itself "abstracts" from documenting the pro-filmic, the extra-cinematic, what the camera is aimed at, into rhythmic fragments and montage. *But*

there are never fragments-of, i.e. of a whole. We are confronted with
the impossibility of adequately lengthy perceptual identification
of the represented. In this film, a *process* made of durations, the
quantity of time, is not sufficient for anything to proceed, here,
as imaginarily communicated space into which one could
somehow identify. The viewer as subject of the content is
made impossible. Rather, the durational sequences become
the subject/object *film* through repetition and the abstract. The
distanciation process inculcated thereby produces a viewer
who him or her self also then no longer can maintain an
anthropormorphic self-identity. Rather, the *film* processes each
"him" and "her," over and over. An equalization takes place
between viewer's processes and film's. Repetition expels identity.

Humanism formulated through film-as-spectacle's anthrop-
omorphisms is here countered. Again the uneasy motoring
of the subject/object; no object is subjected *to* anything; no
subject is instanced (or thereby objectified). The material of
ideology covers all social practices, which, additionally, are *all*
theoretical, and no less real for that.

"Broadly I see structuralism as a result of the dialectical
problem of the concept of order (ordering) in relationship to
experience" (Malcolm LeGrice, "Kren's films," *Studio International*, Film Issue, November 1975, p. 187).

32   The London Filmmakers
Co-operative

Around 1971 the debates at the London Filmmakers Co-
operative were against the mechanistic notion of structure
adumbrated by P. Adams Sitney in his 1969 essay "Structural
film," in *Film Culture*. The London Filmmakers Co-op attempted
dialectical notions of structure which had much more to do
with a radically materialist structuralism, simultaneous with
a post-structuralist critique of mechanistic systems including
any dualistic dialectic itself (whether in social anthropology,
semiotics, or film). It must be recalled that at the Co-op the term

"structure" was used more to refer to films which inculcate in the viewer processes of "attempting to arrest," *attempting* to decipher. Film "as manipulation attempt and awareness thereof" (Gidal, LFMC catalogue, 1969). And "the necessity for the term structur*ing*" (Dunford, Ibid.).[22] "Structuralism can be thought of as a development *from* existentialism,[23] making extreme subjectivity compatible with order by removing from the notion of structure either an *a priori* or an authoritarian implication, the main bases of existential rejection of order. Order is no longer seen as a fixed, immutable condition of the world, but the consequence of changing and developing *acts of ordering*. Whilst there is a recognition that no fixed structure for experience exists, there is also a recognition that there can be no neutral state of unconditioned experience. The development of experience depends on developments of structuring. I see the movement from Cézanne to Analytical Cubism as the historical basis of visual structural art. In 'The Structuralist Activity' Barthes talks of a process whereby the structuralist decomposes the real and then recomposes it. The reconstructed 'object' which I take to imply mainly the structuralist art object, is described as 'intellect added to object.' He stresses that 'between the two objects, or two tenses, of structuralist activity, there occurs *something new* . . .' Structuralist art can be thought of as the material formation of experience through the explicit incursion into the thing or event observed by the mode of observation. In this sense, structuralist art does not *express* experience derived from the world: it *forms* experience in the trace of a dialectic between perceiver and perceived. It is perhaps this concentration on structure as process or activity which most recommends the project to the time-based film medium at the present time" (LeGrice, "Kren's films," op.cit., written 1974).

Such formulations were current from 1970 onwards at the Co-op, and brought issues to bear on the film-practice, and on the way a film could inform the making and theorizing of a *next* work by the same or another filmmaker. This meant that the Filmmakers Co-op had an ongoing public, *social*, definition of practice, as practical as it was theoretical. It was a political necessity for the collective work of the London Filmmakers Co-operative filmmakers; collective was meant to mean such for production, distribution, exhibition and critical/theoretical/polemical work. Precisely because of this materialist and radically socialist notion of the utilization and collectivization of the means of production, and their open access, it was unnecessary to set up a pseudo-collectivity for each specific film. Each film was usually the main work of one filmmaker, but the collective work that went into making that film was always acknowledged in day to day practice as a basis for the process of filmmaking in the first place. That is why, for example, many films made at the London Filmmakers Co-op were printed by or with the help of others than those who shot them; that is why shared information as to grading on the printer, purchasing stock from cheap sources (East German Orwo, for example), testing out effects with a group of five or six filmmakers and discussing these effects whilst still in production, and so on, was commonplace. The kind of collective work engaged in at the Filmmakers Co-op still has not been seriously attempted by more than a few filmmakers or groups, though some deficiencies of the Co-op methods at other levels were recognized and led, for example, to *Four Corners* and *Circles* around 1977, and to changes in male domination at the Co-op (Mary Pat Leece, "Working at the Film Co-op," unpublished tape, 1985).

33   Repetition

The exhaustive, the permutative as the endlessness of the return of the same/seeming same, produces the need (here is where reflexivity comes in) to decipher/arrest the image and structure. Structurings, constantly in process, defence against pre-given meaning, a defensive practice: the process of materialist experimental film-work is the constant movement of eye and brain, contradictions inseparable from the processes of the film as material, and as materialist, i.e. constantly transforming the represented in relation to the operation of the cinematic apparatus and its ideologies. Ideologies of viewing and of the viewed. The dialectic of subject and object. Durations (shots, sequences, *moments* are always simultaneous to constant contradiction between image and filmic representation, meaning and meaning-lessness, "realist" constructs and its ideological. Each film-moment therein being a moment of contradiction, of opposites held only to be simultaneously unheld, *and thereby productive*. This is different from illusionist/narrative production.

Repetition takes you, as subject-viewer, back to attempt to see "what is" and back into, and out from, the process of material-effects-in-film. Constant reification/non-reification forces an inability to make natural *either* of these levels of the cin-ematic. Impossible arrest. The exhaustiveness brought to bear by repetition empties out either side of the contradictorily operative film function. The viewer is thus placed in a space of demeaned, demeaninged cinematicity: attempts at representa-tion, defences against such. The norm for meaning becomes, thereby, non-isolable film-usage: film as materialist social func-tion through the work at hand.

Communication's impossibility; predicated as communication is on the apparatus's transparency and final irrelevance. As a result of (post-)structural/materialist strategies, the viewer is no longer situated as consumer or imaginary producer. The demands of the film-work and the demands of the viewer cannot be seen as congruous or homogenous but in material opposition and subversion. There can be no overdetermination (reductive "end" to (the) matter) of one "part," of either reification or de-reification. No final part, no end to either the filmically given or the part/apart viewer-as-cipher. Very few films "succeed" at any of this. Fail Better. Few films try for the unsuccesses, unpleasures, struggles, resistances; few films are, in short, *practices*.

34   Humanism and anti-humanism[24]

"In 1845, Marx broke radically with every theory that based history and politics on an essence of man. . . . A radical critique of the *theoretical* pretensions of every philosophical humanism. . . . The definition of humanism as an *ideology*.

. . . That there is a universal essence of man (sic) and that this essence is the attribute of each single individual who is its real subject. . . . [So] it is essential that each carries the whole human essence, if not in fact, at least in principle; this implies an *idealism of the essence*. So empiricism of the subject implies idealism of the essence and vice versa. . . . This was replaced . . . by a historico-dialectical materialism of practice (economic practice, political practice, ideological practice, scientific practice) in their characteristic articulations . . . a concrete conception of the specific differences that enable us to situate each particular practice in the specific differences of the social structure." (Althusser reduces, and "forgets" sexuality, does not (want to) understand domestic labour and patriarchal ideology). "For the corollary of theoretical Marxist anti-humanism is the recognition and knowledge of humanism itself: as an ideology. Marx never fell into the idealist illusion of believing that the knowledge of an object might ultimately replace the object or dissipate its existence. . . . Ideology is a system (with its own logic and rigour) of representations (images, myths, ideas, or concepts, depending on the case) endowed with a historical existence and role within a given society. . . . In the majority of cases these representations have nothing to do with "consciousness": they are usually images and occasionally concepts, but it above all as *structures* that they impose on the vast majority. . . . In ideology, people do indeed express, not the relation between them and their conditions of existence, but *the way* they live the relation between them and their conditions of existence. . . .

"The bourgeoisie lives in the ideology of *freedom* the relation between it and its conditions of existence: that is, its real relation (the law of a liberal capitalist economy) but invested in an imaginary relation 'all people are free, including free labourers whom it exploits and is going to exploit in the future'. . . . Ideology as a system of mass representations is indispensable to any society if people are to be formed, transformed, and equipped to respond to the demands of their conditions of existance" (Louis Althusser, "Marxism and humanism," *For Marx*, Allen Lane, The Penguin Press, 1971, pp. 227–35). Men live their relation to the sex class women in precisely the same way, *and* the representations *do* have to do with consciousness as therein (in the former) reside also the oppressive, *real*, meanings which we live; ". . . we must know what patriarchy is in order to understand to what extent it is theoretically independent of capitalism. Only such an understanding can enable us to account for the historical independence of these two systems. Only then is it possible to establish the material basis for the connection between the struggle against patriarchy and the struggle against capitalism" (Christine Delphy, "The main enemy," (1970), *Close to Home*, Hutchinson, London, 1984, p. 75). "What I want is for the author to really override my world view with hers. Otherwise I don't see the point of her making a film. If her production is for me to project my world view onto, I don't need her production to project my world view! . . . Show how a different view is just as real, how it becomes meaning. . . . Show that it is constructed to look *like* reality" (Christine Delphy, " 'On representation and sexual division', Interview with Lisa Cartwright," *Undercut*, no. 14/15, Summer 1985, pp. 19–20).

Anti-humanism is necessary even when not utilized by filmmakers as a conscious concept. Theory often lags behind practice. The machine is a critique of humanism, the cinematic apparatus is durable, in duration, machined, endless, *and* unendurable, in duration, machined, endless. It is the ineffable stare, machined by the projection of film. The stare as machined via the durable/unendurable continuum is produced by the anti-humanistic debodied, desexed, screened image, forcing the productive viewer from impossible consumption. The relation to an anti-humanistic stare, as opposed to some metaphor for the human, is crucial to this concept. It is not "about" the machine representing a machined process; it is *producing* that process in interminable coextensiveness *through* the viewer/cipher. The person as effect, capable of causing other effects, not as itself (himself/herself) originary cause.[25] These anti-humanistic formations of the machine, camera, can go against determinants of current convention as to "what a machine does" or "what a machined stare means."

An example: Rodchenko's photographic machined stare is produced through images taken *against* the convention which states that the photographic camera must be at human height, out into the world. Rodchenko situates a *new* machine, angles of the stare not those of "photography." What we conceive of as, at any historical moment, likeness *to* the machine, is not necessarily that which most precisely *produces* machined anti-humanism, "machine *qua* machine." The automat-photograph which reminds the viewer immediately of the "machine," the photo-booth, in fact produces an amateurist, "natural truth" image which does *not* produce thereby a machined anti-humanistic effect. Thus, what is machinistic depends on the specific interrelations and conjuncture of image, ideology, technology, and the various histories of the subject-cipher, as well as conditions which maintain, or repress, the apparatus (defined to include all elements of film and the cinematic).

35 Socialism/optimism/pessimism

"Well, it would be an idealism to think that a kind of counter-cinema, as some would call it, would somehow finally replace Hollywood. You don't just wipe that out . . . you have to deal in terms of the concrete power relations of who's running Hollywood, what the business and economic interests are. Obviously an avant-garde that sees itself as separately changing things is naive. That's why avant-garde filmmakers *do* have to be socialists, because that cannot happen in a vacuum outside of the economic. I don't go so far as to say that what follows is always true, but certainly the economic and sexual are the kinds of co-determining final instances without whose change all other important change remains unrooted. What won out in the USSR was a kind of economism, which was necessary, industrialization was so important against the West's aggressions that culture, the Soviet avant-garde work of the 1920s, suffered. One can hardly, though, say that the moment wasn't right. One can merely say that the forces of capitalism were always stronger in the end in these revolution-ary historical moments, in this case necessitating Russia's industrial and military defence. We do know that the moment of highest responsiveness to cultural revolution was in times of, and right after, political revolution, in the Soviet Union around 1915–25, during the Bavarian Soviet around 1919, in Cuba after 1959, in Nicaragua after 1979. This is why the entropic position of hopelessness is not decadent. One has neither to be romantic nor idealist about the future.

"   . . . I'm merely less optimistic about everything. It's really part of anti-humanistic Marxism. It doesn't allow humanism which, even on the left, is *always* a bourgeois phenomenon, and that's why so many Marxists who have this idealist hope are very dangerous. You could then (wrongly) overcharacterize this position of mine as 'entropic' and therefore 'trivialization of *all* attempts, all work'. I'm merely saying that any kind of humanistic hopeful *enthusiasm* is a detour from what's necessary.

"You can't really begin to do any concrete material work in your own practice until you believe that everything is hopeless, the way a new film comes from the dead end that the last work produced, and from the dead end not from some shining light the next work is produced. Everything else is just good-conscience stuff. That's the position, not a trivialization of the possibilities of change in the power relations within ideologies and within day to day practices: image, language, economic, and sexual relations. I absolutely think that those kinds of transformations of real political change *can* take place. In relation to film, they might take place in the way that the story-telling and the narrative imaginary aspect of dominant representations might not have that strangle-hold over the way one is constantly situated, and reproduced, consciously and unconsciously, as inevitable. As if one were inevitable to all forms of political power as-is, 'natural', outside of objective, and subjective, *positions*, and positions of resistance" (Peter Gidal, "Politics, history and the avant-garde," *Wide Angle*, vol. 5, no. 2, March 1983, pp. 77 and 76). "One has to distinguish between radical and reactionary pessimism; the latter leads to hyperbolic, metaphoric, Kitsch romanticism, voyeurism, and illusions of change. Reactionary pessimism is like reactionary optimism, you feel so bad you feel good. It's the *Guardian/New Statesman/Village Voice* position basically. You hear enough of the heavy-handed sound-tracks of European male heroes wandering through South and Central America, suffering (in the name of the nameless masses, or for themselves) that you feel so bad at eleven o'clock at night that you feel good. There is also the reactionary pessimism of the decadent movements having had their resurgence in neo-Expressionism and equally in the 'next' phase of film, painting, sculpture, architecture, and writing: 'post modern' pastiche and simulacra in Germany, Italy, and the United States, and somewhat in England though not to the same degree. A materialist position can not be optimistic" (Mike O'Pray, "Gidal interview," *Monthly Film Bulletin*, British Film Institute, London, February 1986).

36   A little polemic on production

All along, the concept of *production* has been utilized in relation to film as materialist process. But the concept "production" on its own does not suffice, for it is open to the query "why production?" and "What is it about production itself that allows it to be given such value for a socialist film-politics? Apart from its being for *use* not *exchange*?"

Perversions of socialist ideology would take from bourgeois artforms not their advanced formulations but their retrograde representational elements. The process of aesthetic production must incorporate the viewer. Capitalist art's ideologies need a capitalist viewer, i.e. a consumer, in order to keep the power of the individual subject ready solely for the reproduction of capital(ism). Patriarchy requires, in its interests, *its* viewer/viewings. The concept of *enjoyment*, as if it were somehow, for "a harmonious moment," outside the political, is a phantasy. So when Godard states "I have given up politics" ("Interview," *The Times*, 22 January 1983), this (and condescension) is evident, as an individual is not in a position to "give up politics" as if it were a choice to *not* have his/her meanings made socially/politically. "Giving up politics" is always a theme of the Right, as are "moral questions 'beyond' politics" (elucidated recently in odes to abjection by Julia Kristeva). Whether one is positioned in productive process through the film and the film through you, or as passive consumer (however much the illusion of superiority *over* the narrative operations holds), whether one thinks one is simply enjoying a consumption or not, whether one knows it is an illusion (Hollywood fictions, Chinese Romances, etc.) or not, the unconscious identifications determine those relations in contradiction to conscious *will*. That is the *locus* of production.

All works are materialist, inasmuch as all social practices are; but use of the term is to define those few that do not suppress or repress this function, the processes of the work at hand, whether it be an aesthetic or social work. Seen rigorously both are both. Smooth functioning of narrative, or of any other social discourse, assumes the suppression/repression of the constructed. Construction verifies the unnaturalness of each practice. So works producing their materialism are materialist; one does not have to read Nietzsche to be positioned as a historical viewer/reader/subject in relation to truth, knowledge, guilt, will, consumption, production, beauty, politics, language! (But it helps.) Moving history forward (history moves forward anyway) is a matter of the new: revolutionary representational systems, all affecting the mass of people. (The only argument *against* that would be a decadent one, that nothing effects anything.) The attempt to construct empty signifiers and non-identities is a process for the production of the political anti-individualist. Hegel posited that "the whole is the identity of identity and non-identity." An advanced *materialist* aesthetic theory of subjectivity could posit no *is*, no being or identity.

The satisfactions in a materialist viewing-process are simultaneously discomforting, a complex of uses not usefulnesses, processes without product, exchanges without calculable profit. Some beauty.

"Labour is the source of all wealth." No, writes Marx, in *Critique of the Gotha Program*, "Nature is just as much the source of use values, and it is surely of such that material wealth consists!" This kind of problem has bearing on production, so as not to fetishize it, and to recall that value is not an *a priori* "good," somehow within moral/ethical categories. "Value" and "production" are important concepts for establishing definitions of what a socialist viewing process that is anti-patriarchal could be; for whom is "value" produced, and so on. What use is the concept of production, if not for the transforming of the relations of production of meaning, and the transforming of class and sex positions, subjective and objective, both both.

37 Autonomy and anonymity

The evictions of narrative, and of any imaginarily present "character" (whether perceptually present or not) can be produced through processes that create filmic anonymity and autonomy. "Simplistically the options of cinematic enunciations might be characterized as *on the one hand* falsely 'neutral', 'omniscient' enunciation of dominant cinema, which poses personality through names of directors, producers, and stars, but which is 'falsely' neutral . . . because its enunciation is that of the hidden cultural ideology expressed through the agents of the production, *and on the other hand* the personal enunciation of the individual film artist. The first option is relatively easy to reject theoretically even if its effects on film practice and structure are difficult to eradicate. However, the problems implicit in the second option and particularly the forms which this has taken on through the New American Cinema practice have been mainly left inarticulate" (LeGrice, "Some notes", op. cit.).

The problematization of subjectivity in contemporary feminist films of Lis Rhodes, Lucy Panteli, Rose Lowder, Joanna Davies, Joanna Millet, Carole Enahoro is a completely different matter. "The American critical tendency, by stressing the film-maker as text, through a continuation of the mythology of romantic individualism, fundamental to the American (potentially genocidal) hero, has helped to re-inforce this 'veering' even where, in another critical framework, other, radical, aspects may have been discernable" (LeGrice, pp. 19–31, op. cit.). "The interpretation becomes inscribed in the forms and devices of work unless dislodged" (op. cit.). Consequently, a general style/code has to be worked against. Some British avant-garde film realizes these necessities, most American, Austrian, German, and French work does not. And when it does, it is opposed even in serious, non-journalistic, film-criticism. The example (again) is Annette Michelson's description of *Wavelength* (1967) as being "a grande metaphor for narrative action" (Annette Michelson, "Toward Snow," *Artforum*, 1971; see also Michelson's "Forward in three letters," *Artforum*, Structural Film Issue, September 1971).

"A hand-held camera, for example, comes to be interpreted as representing the film-maker's subjective vision, and as the culture develops, this inscription of meaning for hand-held camera movement becomes pre-determined – becomes part of 'the language' – and refined in subsequent films within those terms. What must be rejected is narrative as it is understood in conventional cinema *and* broad narrativity as it comes to reappear in experimental film variously through: the replacement of story diegesis by mechanistic structure, the illusion of documentary transparency, particularly under the guise of representing the process of a film's making, and most centrally, narrative as it comes to reappear through any form of anthropomorphic, individualist identification with the filmmaker. The sought-for anonymity for the filmmaker should clearly not be interpreted as a reversion from individual responsibility to the loss of self in the corporate" (LeGrice, "Some notes", op. cit.). The corporate is here to be understood as *opposed* to collectivity.

It is a desire for a relative form of anonymity, "not a superficial anonymity brought into false existence through such things as 'coldness' – heavy atmospheric intervention – which functions precisely in opposition to its supposed intention. Anonymity must in fact be created through transformation dialectically posited into the filmic event itself. That is, anonymity must be the result, at the specific instance; it too must be produced rather than illustrated or obliquely 'given' in a poetical sense." (Gidal, "Theory and definition of structural/materialist film", Film issue, *Studio International*, November 1975 and *Structural Film Anthology* (1976 and 1978, British Film Institute, London).[26]

"Gidal's concept suggests that the anonymity of the filmmaker is achieved primarily through establishing the autonomy of the produced work ('the content thus serves as a function upon which, time and time again, the filmmaker works to bring forth the filmic event') – albeit a work which does not

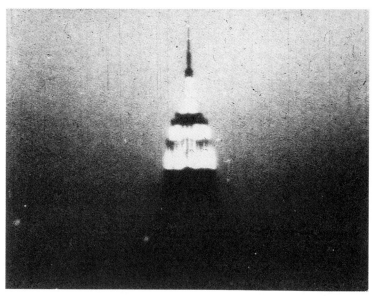

42 Andy Warhol, *Empire* (1963)

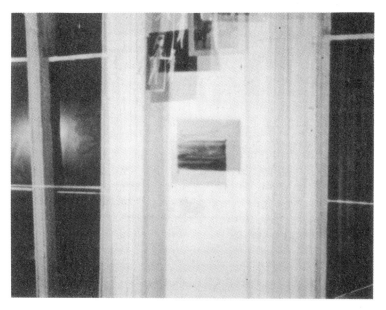

43 Michael Snow, *Wavelength* (1966/7)

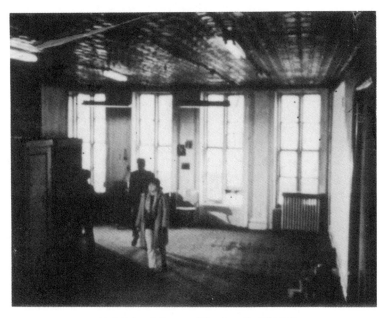

44 Michael Snow, *Wavelength* (1966/7)

efface the traces of its worked-on-ness, and is a work of process. . . . This also opposes the kind of seeming complete autonomy of the physical film object which 'total abstraction' might be thought to offer. The film work presented as a film *work* is an attempt to permit the spectator to utilize, appropriate, transform the film unencumbered by the ego of the filmmaker – its terms are public rather than private – a public discourse . . . to produce a condition for the spectator of response to the film . . . and the spectator's possibility of resistance to the identification with the pleasure of the filmmaker or even resistance to an identification with the filmmaker's act of resistance" (LeGrice, "Some notes", op. cit.).

What I am trying to bring forth is the relation of perceptual mimesis, psychoanalytic narcissism, social narrative phallocracy, and identification, as interminably linked. Identification is inseparable from the procedures of narrative, though not totally covered by them. The teller "needs" the listener, and the latter's empowering – "need" as power *over*. Collusion is with the teller's story, its "necessary" durations, identifications,

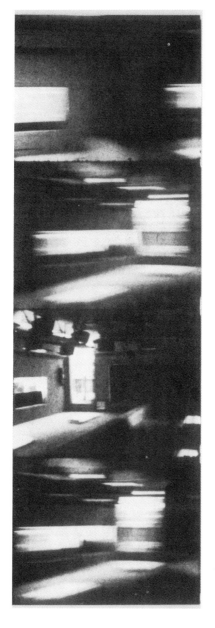

45 Michael Snow, ←——————→ (*Back and Forth*, 1969)

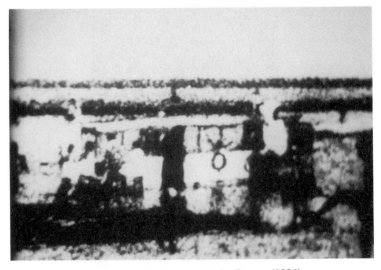

46   Carole Enahoro, *Oyinbo Pepper* (1986)

its needs, given as the Real, and as Truth. As if it could be "beyond" politics, "outside" ideology.

The problematic of anonymity also concerns the question as to whether narrative is structurally mystificatory, resting its "authoritativeness" on that. The fact that it requires identificatory procedures and a lack of distanciation to function, and that its only possible functioning is at an illusionistic level, indicates that the problematic has a resolution. In that sense, *it is more of a problem than a problematic*. Certain technical devices operate in a codified manner, under specific laws, to repress (material) film-time and space, and to suppress the operation of repression itself. Yet what is important here is to not misunderstand this use of the term "repression" as if its opposite were freedom. Repression here is the annihilation of the subject and the material. This is the specific repression polemicized and theorized against. Its opposite would be the de-annihilation of the subject's and the material's processes, processes of autonomy and anonymity.[27]

Radical experimental film is countered by the desire to leave the cinema, in the face of a materialist avant-garde.

Notes

1 With the exception of *The Chelsea Girls*, where each single take is in constant relation to a take on the "other" screen (left *or* right), thus denying any simple verité-ideology. Additionally, each "take" begins, and ends, several minutes in advance of, or after, the other screen's. This allows for reloading of the projectors, and (but) also disallows any pure notion of "begin" and "end," and, therefore, of synchronicity, of any alignment one to the other.

2 "It [the painting] is there, but form is given it without which 'it' is not." Heinrich Wölfflin, *Die Klassische Kunst*, F. Bruckmann-Verlag, Munich, 1904, p. 270.

3 The small, hand-holdable Leica had much to do with this.

4 "The future belongs to the film that cannot be told."

Germaine Dulac, *Le Rouge et le Noir*, July, 1928.

Other useful formulations for film can be eked out:

"For objective dialectics, the absolute is also to be found in the relative. The unity, the coincidence, identity, resultant force, of opposites, is conditional, temporary, transitory, and relative."

Lenin, "On Dialectics", in *Materialism and Empirio-Criticism*,
London, Martin Lawrence, 1938

"If the cinema is to survive it will only be through a few groups refusing to visit commercial kinos and working out their ideas, as Kuleshov did, on paper. They will have to be more avant-garde than the French in 1927, more cut off from equipment than the Russians after the revolution. They will have to attack the formula and not tolerate it; they must learn to walk out from pictures that however technically perfect are based upon false ideas. They will have to make scraps of film that every commercial producer would refuse and project them on kitchen walls before small groups determined to tear them to pieces."

Bryher (Winifred Ellerman), "The Hollywood code II", *Close Up*, December, 1931, London and Territet.

"The European filmmakers certainly made much the strongest impression . . . though without the presence of clearly established masters. But that's a way of thinking which many of the Europeans reject. . . . It's difficult to pin down, but one senses an attitude towards filmmaking not as the production of certain great works but as an ongoing motive of artistic work. . . . European filmmakers are wary of the structure and ideology which might create the conditions for cultural imperialism in the area of filmmaking. They are, therefore, involved in a redefinition of the nature and function of filmmaking that differs from those of the Americans who are making their way gradually towards the centre of our own culture."

P. Adams Sitney, talking with Annette Michelson, "A conversation on Knokke and the independent filmmaker", *Artforum*, May, 1975.

5 (a) More, equals desire, equals desire for, equals desire for *more*.

(b) " . . . direct challenge to the founding difference of the representation of subjects, men and women" relies, unfortunately on pre-given, therefore naturalized, signifieds and referents. What goes against this is a *positioning* as radically asexual, its constant conflict with the histories of the viewer/subject, not defined by "the sexual" or the sexuality of gender. This is *not* a voluntarist positing of an "un-founded" (i.e. simply neither male nor female) subject.

(c) Although Laura Mulvey's crucial essay "Visual pleasure and narrative cinema" dealt with the latter form of film (and incorporated acknowledged lessons from experimental film), she later took up some issues of the avant-garde explicitly:

"The slippage of the there and the not-there, the trying to form things, produces suspense. . . . I find *Condition of Illusion* very fascinating, very involving and very pleasurable to watch. . . . There is a kind of natural tendency of the spectator to form a narrative internally or externally, whether the film-maker wants you to or not, which is a way in which the object up there on the screen escapes possible intention. . . . I wanted to point out against the often-held view that this is not pleasurable, that there is a certain pleasure in the eruption of the apparatus . . . the marking of the apparatus, the underlining of the focus/de-focus which has a pleasurable side and which brings us back to fascination too."

Laura Mulvey, "Discussion on technology, ideology, and the avant garde", *The Cinematic Apparatus*, op. cit., p. 166–7.

6 Mike Dunford, "Experimental/avant-garde/revolutionary/film practice," *After Image*, no. 6, Summer 1976.

7 A personal note. When criticized by some filmmakers at the
   London Film Co-op at Robert Street (1969–70) for not helping with
   the physical labour of building (e.g.) the projection-booth, etc, my
   retort was that all my concentration was on making films. Eight
   months later (or 18?) it sunk in – we all had as filmmakers to do
   both, and it did, from then on, seem equally ludicrous to me when
   others refused physical labour when we moved to and built up the
   Prince of Wales Crescent site.

8 In individualist interpretive writing (whether criticism or fiction),
   giving itself as historical truth, much must be subsumed to "the
   literary," to the metaphor, to the *as if*, or *like*. Musil's *The Man
   without Qualities*, for a contrary example, utilizes this endless
   metaphorizing to the point of exasperation, simultaneous to a
   subjectivist endlessness, rather than as ostensible substantiation.

9 It must be noted that the term deconstruction is here meant in very
   opposition to Burch's definition, taken from Metz and Derrida, as
   Annette Kuhn here utilizes it outside of the notion of strict
   cinematic codes which would then be, each time, negated or
   deconstructed. She uses the term to posit the *constant* denial of
   meaning whilst simultaneously attempted reproduction of images
   is effected, by the cinematic apparatus, camera, editing, lighting,
   speed, grain, and so on.

10 In recent film and art criticism "transformation" has been
   reappropriated for its transcendental ideology – the anti-materialist
   dialectic.

11 "Loyalty is the theme as Roy Cohn feasts friends," *New York Times*,
   1 July 1983. "What brought them there was loyalty . . . on the
   guest list were Andy Warhol, Carmine G. De Sapio, Calvin Klein,
   and Abraham Beame . . . conservatives and liberals. . . . 'You
   mention Roy Cohn (Joe McCarthy's leading council in the 1950s
   anti-communist witchhunts) and some people almost want to tear
   your throat out. It makes you want to stand up and say I don't care
   about McCarthy or anyone else. I know Roy Cohn and I swear by
   him. The quality of his friendship is exquisite. He still wears the
   label 'McCarthyite' with pride . . .'. The most ringing tribute came
   from Stanley M. Friedman, the Bronx Democratic chairman and Mr
   Cohn's law partner at Saxe, Bacon and Bolan: ' . . . this party, and
   the friends of Roy Cohn, shall forever live.' " Cohn died in 1986;
   Friedman is in jail for fraud, not for his prose.

12 Nancy Woods, on Lis Rhodes' *Light Reading*. This essay's history
   betrays the pretentiousness of certain critics. After requiring

changes and rewrites, and then "thinking it over for a year," Constance Penley and another member of the editorial board of *Camera Obscura* rejected the article. *After Image* (Simon Field) wanted it for a phantasmatic British Avant-Garde Film issue. Then a *Derek Jarman* issue came out instead. *Undercut* in turn was delighted to print the article, even had it typeset, but by then Nancy Woods felt that as it was nearly three years old it had to be reworked, something she had planned previously to do in conjunction with *After Image*. She was then happy to let the essay stand as-is for *Circles* to use as program notes, and it is from such, finally, that these quotes are taken.

13 For an excellent critique of Snow's work, see Kip Turner, "Letter on Snow," in *Ideolects*, no. 13, 1983.

14 Esther Shub co-wrote the shooting script for Eisenstein's *Strike* "There is a resemblance of the long tracking shot in the factory, in her film *The Fall of the Romanov Dynasty* (1927), a superb compilation film, to the one in *Strike*" (Jay Leyda, "Lecture, Collective for Living Cinema," 6 March 1983). At this screening/ lecture, sixty-five people attended; by the time the film had been shown, and *before* the lecture proper, twenty-four people were left. Half a century and the work is still deemed too difficult and

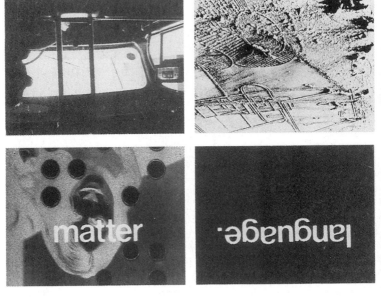

47   Peter Gidal, *Upside-Down Feature* (1967–72)

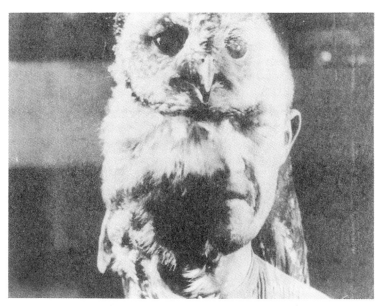

48 Sergei Eisenstein, *Strike* (1925)

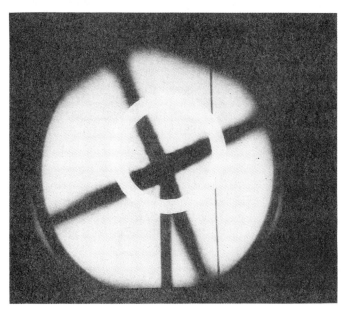

49 Sergei Eisenstein, *Strike* (1925)

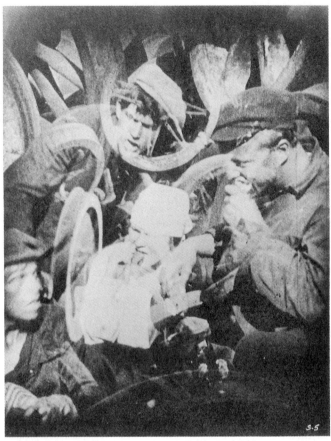

50 Sergei Eisenstein, *Strike* (1925)

abstruse even in a space set up for non-commercial and non-
mainstream film. "There's very little footage left from 1917 of
Moscow so there's some repetition" (ibid.). The Shub film is edited
together sequentially, whilst at the same time it is so obviously
"newsreel-type" footage that it is always also a *construction*. "It
feels real, feels like in spite of the obvious compilation that that
was the way things were, how they looked. The 1913 war footage
had the most leeway and laxness, planes that weren't even
invented yet were shown, and so on. Some repeats of members of
the Provisional Duma Council were because no other footage
existed, but not out of irony" (ibid.). The titles about soldiers being

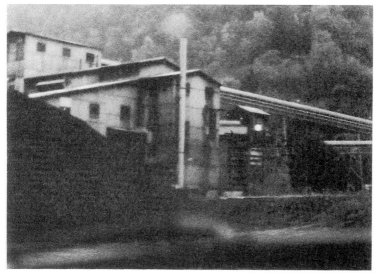

51 Bill Brand, *Coalfields* (1984)

cannon-fodder were placed in such a way that when seeing images
of men going to war one remembered those previous titles, thus
the propaganda was undermined, whilst at the same time the truth
of the propaganda, the need to fight imperialism, remained. What
it thus did was de-sentimentalize war. The long tracking shot to
the right, in a factory, as in *Strike*, gives both more "truth" to the
documented surroundings and more "subjectivity" to the apparatus, less "objectivity". (Thus a different kind of truth.) And the
way the film is montaged or edited together by Shub lets many
sequences take their time, static shots in formal relation to
nonstatic, so that "the shot" is often not dominated by "events"
depicted. Shub's importance and influence have still not been dealt
with. "She was very careful about whose work, what specific
images, she used in her compilation films" (ibid.).

Bearing on both Shub's and Eisenstein's work: There exists a
letter from Beckett to Eisenstein which acknowledges precisely that
the script, as was the scenario, is "a function of the means of
realization" (Samuel Beckett, 3 February 1936). The letter's veracity
has been verified by Leyda, Beckett, and Naum Kleiman in Moscow.

15 My problem would be with the plausible coherence of time/space
relationships.

16 This book/catalogue, *A Perspective on English Avant-Garde Film*, was
published also in English/German, and English/French editions.

The show (covering 1966–76) travelled to thirty cities in twelve countries over a two-year period. It is *not* to be confused with the Arts Council/Hayward Gallery "Perspectives on British avant garde film" (looseleaf catalogue, for the films accompanying the exhibition (and catalogue) *Film as Film 1910–1975*). Now you know. And *The Elusive Sign* which is travelling in 1988–1990 to approximately twenty countries consists of five experimental film and four video programmes representing 1977–1987.

17 "Reproduction held into a representation" in Stephen Heath's useful (and wonderful!) formulation from 1977. *Against Reproduction* is still the political necessity.

18 *Where*, and *what*, in *Yes No Maybe Maybe Not*, could be conceived of (or seen) as beginning and end? There is no adequacy deducible *from* the perceived *to* such a conception (or knowledge). Analogously, whether the representations of water/Battersea towers, is, finally, iconic (approximation of the real world) or indexical (link to the real world) does not matter: the montage is to disallow meaning to be solidified from the non-integratedness of the "two" images, their montage-sequencing, repetition, overlap, condensation, and lack of reconstruction *towards*. The illusionist capture of time, representing the present, necessitates an illusionist structure to effect that, and this film is the opposite of that necessity! The constantly attempted re-arrestation attempt forces a work careful in the disparity between the seen and the known, a constant construction *from* the material. As such. anything represented is always already the pro-filmic of *this* film, not some imaginary pro-filmic history outside, "adequately portrayed" and then "worked upon."

19 In opposition to film as material we have, for example, Gilles Deleuze's *Cinema, The Movement-Image* (Athlone Press, 1986). It is idiotic when French humourless philosophers discourse on film, elevating the commonplace and the commonsensical as if *The Diary of a Nobody* hadn't been written. How to define "movement-image"? Deleuze's answer: "As mother." When it comes to the empirical to back up his notions about cinema and time with respect to *Wavelength*, Deleuze sees "some girls coming to listen to the radio, they hear a man climb the stairs and collapse to the floor, but the zoom has already passed him, giving way to one of the girls." This teleological fairy-tale is laughable. After this act of not seeing he happily analyses the events "in temporal and philosophical terms," ending with a call for a "radical cinematic practice à la Hitchcock". Further derogatory hysteria occurs to give the semiotics of film a "philosophical" backup: "At a certain point I try to show that phallocentrism and feminism are tantamount to the same thing" (Jacques Derrida, in *Critical Exchange*

17, Winter, 1985, p. 31). "Feminism is nothing but the operation of a woman who aspires to be like a man. Feminism too seeks to castrate. It wants a castrated woman" (Derrida, *Semiotexte*, vol. III, no. 1, 1978, p. 130). As a proper deconstructionist, Derrida needs to perpetuate, amongst other things, biological categories.

20 Identification: "Mental mechanism whereby the individual attains gratification, emotional support, or relief from stress by consciously or unconsciously attributing to him/herself the characteristics of another person or a particular group" (*Websters New Collegiate Dictionary*). Identification also causes a great deal of anguish! Against sexual identity would be, then, neither "difference" (woman-as-other *vis-à-vis* a (male) norm, outside language and power) nor "sameness" (woman-as-same, taking (assimilating or complementing) the (male) role in patriarchy, identifying with it, such a role denying women's subjective and objective histories and powers). Both "woman-as-other" and "woman-as-same" would be conceptualizations of description *and* prescription, due to ideological reproduction-in-language. *And* woman does not take into account women.

The concept of *sexual* difference is one figuration upon which one group asserts its power, another its opposition. Revolutionary would be to not be defined by the sexual. It comes down to the right of sexlessness, the non-fetish as woman (and man), rather than the right to *be* "a woman" or "a man". The material positioning through anti-patriarchal theatrics is the situating of viewer–listener *against* the grain of patriarchal authority (politics), drive (psychoanalysis) and signified (culture).

21 Although the filming situation is narrow in this film, being confined to five short sequences all filmed from within a dock-side cafe, the work does not aim to be a homologue of the space-time relations intrinsic to the situation and procedure of the filming itself. The filmed sequences are largely separated from their representational function, to become the subject of subsequent systematization, where their relationships within the film-presentation are much more significant than the procedural relationship with their origin (yet) the broad effect and historical significance of this film lies in shifting the emphasis of structural activity away from the filmmaker's ordering of the filmic subject to that of the spectator's structuring of the filmic presentation. The film's viewer must engage in a speculative, reflexive structuring of the film as it proceeds. The five sequences are sufficiently similar to each other to ensure that the initial problem faced is the discrimination of the shots themselves" (Malcolm LeGrice, "Kren's Films," *Studio*

International, Film Issue, November 1975, p. 187). "I would quote *TV* as the first thoroughly realized work of reflexive cinema, transferring the primary arena for the structuralist activity to the viewer of a film itself" (ibid.).

22 Whilst some of us lagged in language, the filmworks were much less mechanistic than their American counterparts, more concerned with a dialectical relation of viewer/film/text as a constant film-as-projected *"problematic of representation through representation"* (Malcolm LeGrice, "On *Room Film 1973*," *Studio International*, 1974). Dunford's formulation of structur*ing* was not unrelated to his and LeGrice's readings of Piaget, which afforded the London filmmakers and theoreticians a way out of the mechanistic, whilst at the same time out of the romantic American model. Roger Hammond's adumbrations crossed those of Dunford in their perpetual relation between filmic articulation and pseudo-scientificity exposed as such viz. *Erlanger Program* (1972), *Klien's Phenomenon* (1973). The spelling is not a misprint. Relevant were his notes on these and other films, his insistence on *non-wholistic*, structured-and-structuring anti-positivism. Hammond's critique was of British empirical philosophy, plenty of which he had to endure at Cambridge, as did John DuCane, prior to working at the Co-op. Their positions preceded by a decade *Screen*'s intimations that perhaps all was well neither with that particular disease, nor with cinema (though *Screen* never did intervene to end it). That Dunford, Hammond, DuCane, so concerned with verbal formulation, were all filmmakers who produced sophisticated, aesthetically advanced works, helped make (with Eatherley, Nicholson, Crosswaite, and a dozen others) for a productive context the likes of which had only existed this century in the 1920s in the Soviet Union. Most of the filmmakers around the London Filmmakers Co-op had art college backgrounds, and were ("additionally") autodidacts of the highest order. It is in this context that the statement, "Broadly I see Structuralism as a result of the dialectic problem of the concept of order/ordering in relation to experience" must be understood, and understood as having been understood at the time 1967–75.

"Kren's first structuralist film then is 3/60 *Bäume im Herbst* (*Trees in Autumn*, 1960), incidentally the first film in general I would call structuralist. Its structuralism is a result of the application of a system, not to subsequent montage of material already filmed with an unconstrained subjectivity, but to the act and event of filming itself. This limitation, by narrowing the space and time range of the shot material, gives rise to a greater integrity in the film as homologue" (LeGrice, op. cit.). Issue is taken with a continuing concern of LeGrice's, namely "integrity," its ethical meanings, but even in its non-normative use as some sort of one-ness, clinically described. This problem occurs again years later in *Undercut* (No. 1, March/April 1981) wherein LeGrice explicates that the term is purely descriptive as in *integral*.

"In *Bäume im Herbst*, the new space/time fusion of the experience of branches shot against the sky IS the plasticity of the shooting system become the relations of the objects; – shots, and their space/time observational relations are inseparable. Structural process becomes object. [I think subject would be more correct here.] This prefigures Snow's *Back and Forth* (1969) and echoes the plasticity of the time/space in a Giacometti" (LeGrice, op. cit.). I would add Barthes' "structure is the residual deposit of duration." At that time, Barthes was of some interest because of the cultural critiques, for example in relation to Brecht, which could be theorized by filmmakers to make more precise what their work might have been attempting or not attempting, rather than as some model to be illustrated. This is why the irrelevancy thereafter of Barthes' work to film-*production* became clear to the Co-op filmmakers by 1975, at a time when his work was just beginning to show major signs of influence on the independent critics revolving around *Screen*, *Artforum*, and *October*. (Stephen Heath got to Barthes (or Barthes to Heath) earlier – by 1969 – he was always ahead of the rest at *Screen*; in early, out late.) If theory *can* precede practice, nevertheless in the case of experimental and avant-garde film in Britain in the period 1966–86, and in political history, the converse has continually been the case.

23 Viennese formal film. "In the case of the combination of existential message and material message form, it is interesting to note how the expressive concept of montage has become a narrative concept. This transition marks the point of departure for the crucial shift made by the Viennese formal film, as . . . it is the films of the Russian Formalists Eisenstein and Vertov which on the whole still followed a narrative form interspersed, as it were, with moments of montage. In Kubelka's and Radax's *Mosaik im Vertrauen* (1950) the film maintains throughout a montage-structure. Montage no longer only serves the sequentially limited articulation of meaning as is the case in the notion of 'expressive concept', but extends to include the whole film: all parts of the film inter-relate. The sound/image montage of Vertov, especially, was a determining factor in this. The courses set were in fact theses: either to carry over the overall structure of the montage into the small organisms of the work, in which case even the tiniest part (that is to say, the

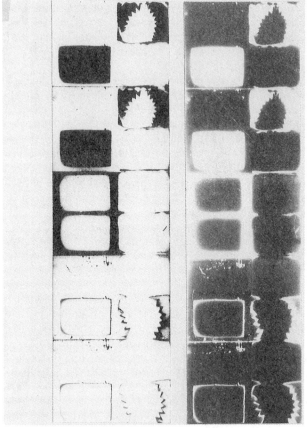

52 David Crosswaite, *Film Number One* (1971)

single frame) obeys a formal law, so that moreover the narration (paradoxically!) is lost (as is curiously the case with the process of permutation, which contributed to the discovery of the twelve-tone row-technique in music, and later to its dissolution) *or* montage itself becomes a form of narration. It is clearly the case that narrative montage keeps the expressive alive, whilst small-scale minimal montage becomes so compressed that the montage itself disappears; montage is transformed into row-technique (seriality). Kubelka, under influence of Webern – speaking formally, technically, and in an abbreviated form (with all its correspondingly partial validity) – transferred and applied twelve tone techniques to

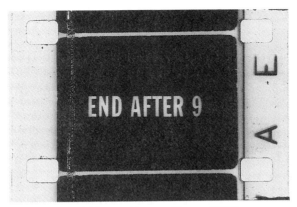

53 Fluxus Group, *Fluxus* (1963)

film – a constellation obviously more probable and more typical for Vienna than for Paris or Hamburg. As context and background for the three purely formal films of Kubelka (*Adebar*, *Schwechater*, *Arnulf Rainer* . . . all of which were found by the British structural/materialist filmmakers of some use, though of less interest than Kren's work) I see a double tradition: that of the Viennese School of music, and that of Eggeling, Vertov, and Dreyer. Vertov was the strictest Russian Formalist, who had already posited a frame-by-frame style of 'film-writing': 'Film writing is the art of writing with film frames' (Vertov). Vertov it was who 'edited the film as a whole' and who, in diametrical opposition to Eisenstein, chose to ignore the route of mise-en-scène in his search for the 'Kinogram'. Many of Vertov's maxims were directly taken over by Kubelka [but not his socialism], such as 'Material-artistic elements of motion – provided by the intervals, the transitions from one movement to another, but not by movement itself'. This 'interval theory' of film of course easily connects with an interval theory of music. Kubelka similarly took over Vertov's equations of image-and-sound relationships as *the* articulations of meaning in film" (Peter Weibel, "The Viennese formal film," *Film as Film*, Arts Council of Great Britain, Hayward Gallery, 1979, p. 110).

Quoting from an unpublished manuscript by a friend of Kubelka's, Weibel writes, quoting, " 'The serial principles of construction, the twelve tone technique of Schoenberg, the twelve tone pieces by Hauer, the extreme frugality of Anton Webern's music, the pictorial effects of Mondrian and the novels of James Joyce were in many respects the starting points for Viennese art

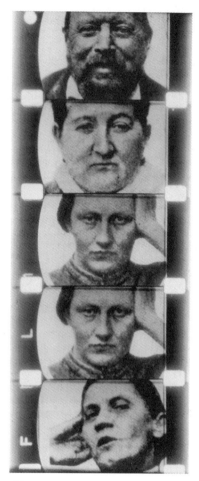

54   Kurt Kren, *48 Heads from the Szondi Test* (1960)

after 1945 and in particular direct preconditions of the films of Kubelka.' Filmic time was conceived as 'measurable' in the same way as musical time; tones as 'time points' became the frames of film. Just as Webern reduced music to the single tone and the interval so Kubelka reduced film to the film-frame and the interval between two frames. Just as the law of the row and its four types determined the sequence of tones, pitches, etc, so now it was the sequence of frames, and of the frame count (phrases in Vertov's terminology), positive and negative, timbre, emotional value, silence, etc; between these factors as in serial music the largest numbers of relationships were produced. *Adebar* (1957) is the first pure Viennese formal film to be generated by these considerations, and perhaps under the influence of Duchamp, Len Lye (the great animator for the British post office!) and other historical pioneers of the 'absolute graphic film' " (Weibel, op. cit., pp. 110–11).

"Extraordinarily, 1960, the year of *Arnulf Rainer* (made of solely black and transparent shots) not only marked the end and highpoint of a distinct development, but also introduced, with Kurt Kren's *48 Heads from the Szondi Test* a new development which might be seen at a superficial glance as a repetition of the first. Kren knew Kubelka's films. Indeed, he had completed his first film *Experiment with Synthetic Sound* as long ago as 1957. But an essential change in tendency must not be overlooked, namely, from a musical structuring to a perceptual. The very title of the second 1960 film refers to an experiment in the psychology of perception. The tendency towards the abstraction of graphic solutions in the domain of formal organization, as it culminated for instance in the abstract light play of *Arnulf Rainer* is here rejected. The succession of photographs (in a realistic style) in *48 Heads from the Szondi Test* (Kren), is not meant to analyse motion or to synthetically simulate it, but to refer to perception itself and the psychic mechanisms which accompany it. It is therefore a subject-oriented and not, as formerly, an object-oriented process" (Weibel, op. cit., p. 112). It becomes, precisely *subject/object*.

"*Unsere Afrikareise* is so disturbing because Kubelka doesn't acknowledge his own position. It's as if he's outside of both cultures or has distanced himself from what he's saying and what he's representing. I'm very suspicious of films which use images which contain potentially horrific meaning and provide a form of play which is intended to somehow overcome that, the idea that you have to go beyond irony and sophistication and make it even

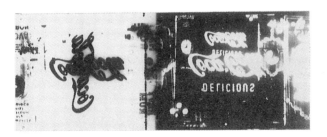

55 David Crosswaite, *Choke* (Double-Screen) (1971)

nore sophisticated, that this will provide an ironic twist. Every film must face up to the range of meanings that can be created" (Weibel, op. cit., p. 18).

What must be finally stated too is that Kubelka's few works have gained, via their association with already assimilated musical concepts, an absurd overvaluation, especially in the United States and France, making *Arnulf Rainer* and *Schwechater* no less extraordinary.

24 "The context for films which e.g. allowed *Wavelength* to find enthusiasm at the Knokke Experimental Film Festival in 1967 exists; a context, namely, within a history of an integration of what could generally be called a *surrealist* aesthetic, congruent with Belgian painting and French surrealist theory. In such a context, *Wavelength* could be re-contextualized, as was, at the following Knokke Festival in 1974, Tsunea Nakai's *Alchemy*. *Alchemy*, with a droning soundtrack and a long-shot fairly wide-angle out in the ghosts-of-wheelbarrows-and-skeletons-of-deserted-warehouses-land, functions as a mask for what is essentially a horror story, a tale of alienated loneliness, bicycle standing dead centre frame (mid-distance), some old rags hanging from the fender blowing (like puffballs) in the wind. The cameraman is the deserted fragment of humanity, absent from the representation but forcefully present as imaginary referent, quite clearly *there* as well. The film is a traditional story 'of hypnotic, isolated, heat-ridden desperation'. But it is, as mentioned, masked. People kept calling it 'that Wavelength film' because of the sound-track's similarity to the former's, and because the forty-five minute film takes a slow zoom from described wide-angle to full close-up on a light bulb slightly behind and above the centre-frame bicycle. The light becomes sharp-edged as the f/stop is closed down; becomes blurry as the f/stop is opened up; there are superimpositions of negative on positive, creating momentary bas-relief. There are also negative shots pure and simple, wherein the distant (and less and less distant) light source is in material presence a flat *black* spot of radiating 'light.' The film does not work with such technical functions as synchronicity, relations between negative and positive in terms of the materialized time-disjunction, etc. (contrary to

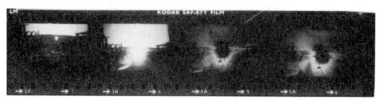

56 Tsunea Nakai, *Alchemy* (1974)

LeGrice's *Yes No Maybe Maybe Not*). The film as potent signifier, potent signified. Post-Hiroshima. Blinding hypnosis. But because of its grandiose scale, its persistent slow zoom, its concentration on a narrow range of effects and operations, it takes on a clarity at least that separates it from the quasi-surrealist meanderings of the other films at the festival, which were still *held* by the Belgian surrealist view of the late 1940s. It comes to mind that the reason so many mediocre phantasies were taken into this festival is precisely that the selection jury's categories of criteria, even those present since 1949, have always been the surrealist shock aesthetic, and that American underground and 'personal' poetic cinema happened, in the fifties and early sixties, to fit this conception through precisely this misreading of for example Jack Smith, Stan Brakhage, Gregory Markopoulos, not to mention Maya Deren and Kenneth Anger. Thus, the American films at that time which made Knokke seem advanced, had slipped into a gap in knowledge. The films were a simulacrum. *Wavelength*, then, because of its incredible shock at the time, also *easily* fitted into this essential misreading, and led to a totally unified final selection jury giving it the grand prize. All this is not to say that no surrealisms are detectable in any of the above-mentioned films, but their thrust (for want of a more adequate word) was certainly not dominantly in that direction nor were their philosophical implications (as they are called) of the surrealist order. The flicker at the end of *Alchemy* takes the film into empty screen, pure brightness of flickering projector light. But in fact, we have a loaded signification for transcendence, for precisely the supposed 'alchemy' of the mind in its transition from materiality to spirituality. The catharsis of this high-pitched drone in conjunction with (i.e. false naturalisation of) the blinkering flashes of light is the Aristotelian theatre all over again. The film is thoroughly retrograde, and it is only unfortunate that such a strong film does not work in an aesthetic that is ideologically productive of anti-illusionist materialism instead of obfuscation and expressionistic story in its simplest, though somewhat masked, form" (Peter Gidal, "On Knokke Experimental Film Festival 1974/5," *Studio International*, March 1975). Such polemico-critical writing virtually forced theory, or at least defence.

25 The unconscious which is the trace and the history of repressions operating socially through individual subjects is also a process, to which there is (outside of idealism) no "opposite" known as "unrepression." The unconscious thus is constantly formed and has its ideological histories. The politics of its sociality can never be separated from specific effects of power. And resistance: unsuppressions and unoppressions.

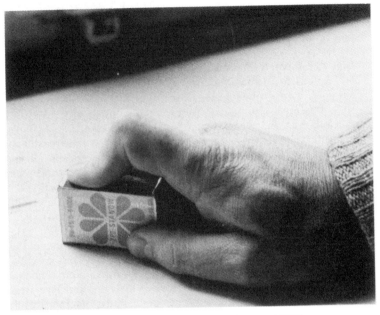

57 Wojciech Bruszewski, *Match Box* (1975)

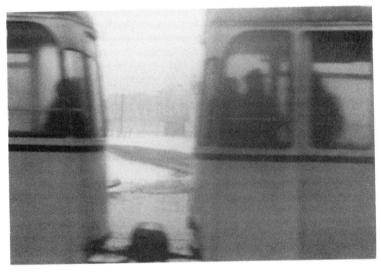

58 Mary Pat Leece, *Mary Voice* (1988)

26 Translations Berlin 1977, Milan 1980, and in Li You Zheng, *Western Film Theories* (1988, Beijing, China).

27 Men and women as *same* (against identities) is a historical revolutionary possibility because radical transformations would be necessary AND that state cannot yet even be conceived, though spoken. Nor could it ever be conceived without (power) struggles. A realm of the aesthetic must equally be the struggle for radical political/ideological transformation of meaning and position.

Materialist anti-representation always is in struggle *with* representation.

Index